FATTY LIVER AND CIRRHOSIS DIET COOKBOOK FOR BEGINNERS

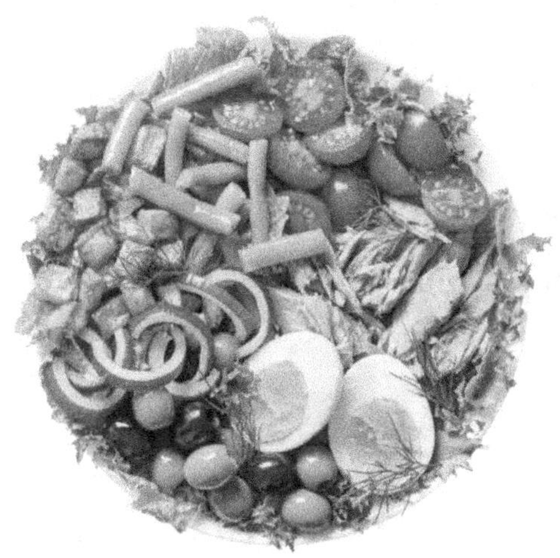

Nourishing Meals and Transformative Nutrition Strategies to Reverse Liver Damage and Improve Wellness

Joan G. Milone

Copyright © 2024 by Joan G. Milone
All rights reserved.

This book is written as a source of information only. The information contained in this book is provided in good faith and is believed to be accurate and reliable as of the date of publication. The author does not assume any responsibility for any errors or omissions that may appear.

HOW TO USE THIS BOOK

1. **Familiarize Yourself.** Begin by going through the booklet to get a feel for the recipes and ingredients. Pay close attention to the beginning parts, which describe the fundamentals of the fatty liver and cirrhosis diet, including which foods to include and avoid.

2. **Plan Your Meals:** Select recipes that meet your nutritional needs and interests. Look for foods with liver-friendly components such as leafy greens, lean meats, healthy grains, and

low salt. Plan your weekly meals, emphasizing diversity and balance.

3. **Gather Ingredients:** Make a shopping list depending on the recipes you choose. Prioritize fresh fruits, lean meats, and whole grains above processed meals and high fats. Stock up on liver-friendly foods such as fruits, vegetables, and low-sodium spices.

4. **Follow Recipes:** Cook according to the cookbook's directions, paying attention to portion quantities and preparation procedures. Include liver-boosting ingredients like garlic, turmeric, and olive oil in your recipes. Experiment with several recipes to keep your meals interesting.

5. **Monitor and Adjust:** Keep note of how your body reacts to the diet, noting any improvements in liver health or overall well-being. Consult a healthcare practitioner if you need help managing your condition. Continue to use the cookbook as a helpful resource for following a liver-friendly diet.

SCAN TO ACCESS MORE AMAZING COOKBOOKS FROM JOAN

Table of Contents

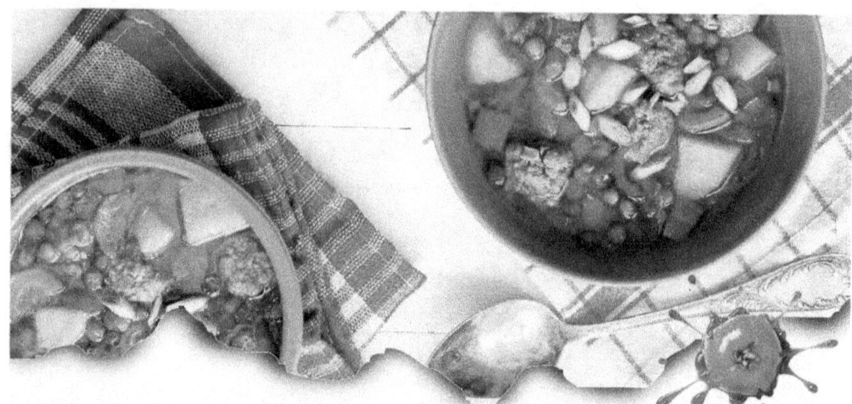

FATTY LIVER AND CIRRHOSIS

DIET COOKBOOK

for Beginners

Nourishing Meals and Transformative Nutrition Strategies
to Reverse Liver Damage and Improve Wellness

With **30 Days** Meal Planner

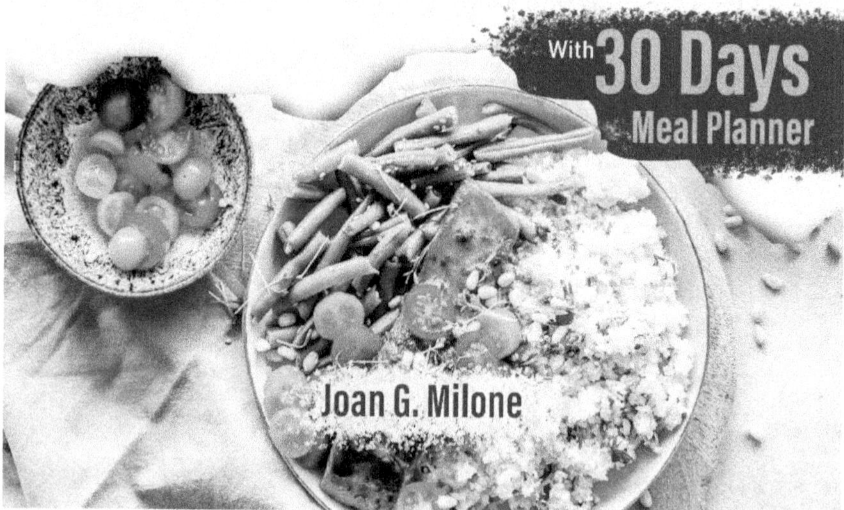

Introduction

In the soft embrace of early morning, where each sunbeam promises a fresh beginning, my kitchen serves as a haven of hope and transformation. This narrative, engraved into the pages of this cookbook, began on a day much like any other, except for the life-altering news that transpired. The diagnosis was clear: a road to restore my liver had to begin. At that time, my kitchen seemed like a new land, full of uncertainty and unspoken inquiries.

But while I stood there, in the silent confusion of my thoughts, an understanding gradually dawned on me. This wasn't simply a challenge; it was a unique opportunity to rethink my relationship with food and investigate its therapeutic properties. This cookbook captures the spirit of that journey, weaving together foods that served as stepping stones to recovery and well-being.

Each dish in this book is more than just a collection of ingredients; they are stories of perseverance and discovery. From the revitalizing simplicity of a fruit-infused drink to the soothing embrace of a substantial vegetable stew, these meals are designed to nurture both the body and the spirit.

I recall well the first recipe that represented a turning point in my wellness journey: a dish that was both simple and meaningful. This culinary innovation taught me a valuable lesson: eating for health does not have to mean sacrificing taste and enjoyment. Rather, it introduces you to a universe in which each taste and ingredient plays an important role in a bigger tale of health and joy.

This cookbook is intended for anybody going on a similar journey, whether they are just getting started or are already on their way. It's a compilation of recipes, experiences, and thoughts that will help you rediscover the joy of cooking and eating while being healthy.

Herein lies more than simply recipes; you'll find tales of optimism, practical knowledge, and a fresh perspective on what it means to eat properly. This book will demonstrate that a health-conscious diet may also be rich, gratifying, and tasty.

Please join me on this wonderful voyage. Let's go through these pages, cook with passion, and appreciate each meal as a kind of self-care and celebration. Welcome to a journey in which the kitchen evolves into a refuge of healing, exploration, and gastronomic joy. Welcome to a new chapter in your life, one tasty meal at a time.

Understanding Cirrhosis and Fatty Liver Disease

Cirrhosis and fatty liver disease, while diverse, share a similar thread: both disorders represent the liver's path from health to discomfort. The liver, the body's quiet worker, is responsible for a variety of processes, including detoxification, metabolism, and nutrition storage. When this critical organ fails, the repercussions can be far-reaching.

Fatty liver disease arises when fat accumulates in the liver cells. It is frequently associated with obesity, diabetes, and high cholesterol, although it can also affect those who do not have these risk factors. This disorder, which appears to be benign at first, can gradually worsen into a more serious illness. In its more severe form, Non-Alcoholic Steatohepatitis (NASH), fat accumulation is accompanied by inflammation and liver cell destruction, paving the way for subsequent difficulties.

Cirrhosis, on the other hand, is the outcome of long-term, ongoing liver damage, which can be caused by a variety of factors such as persistent alcohol consumption, hepatitis, or fatty liver disease. It denotes a stage of severe liver injury, marked by scarring (fibrosis) and the creation of regenerating nodules. This scarring changes the liver's structure and function, reducing its capacity to digest nutrients, hormones, medicines, and poisons. Cirrhosis can progress to liver failure, which is a potentially fatal illness.

Understanding these disorders is critical since their early stages frequently go unreported because they do not produce symptoms. When symptoms occur, they may include tiredness, weakness, and weight loss. As the condition continues, more serious symptoms such as jaundice, swelling in the legs and abdomen, and disorientation may develop, indicating severe liver damage.

The silver lining is the possibility of prevention and treatment. Lifestyle adjustments, particularly in food and exercise, are critical in treating and, in many cases, reversing the early stages of fatty liver disease and reducing the advancement of cirrhosis. This emphasizes the significance of early identification and proactive health decisions in maintaining liver health.

Dietary Considerations for Liver Health

Diet is essential for maintaining liver health. The liver, an organ proficient at regeneration and adaptability, responds astonishingly to intelligent dietary choices. Understanding the influence of nutrition is critical for persons with liver disorders such as cirrhosis or fatty liver disease, as well as everyone who wants to keep their liver healthy.

A liver-friendly diet emphasizes complete, unadulterated foods while maintaining balance and moderation. Fruits and vegetables, which are high in antioxidants and important nutrients, form the foundation of this diet. These components aid in the fight against inflammation and protect liver cells from harm. Leafy greens, in particular, are useful because they aid in detoxifying processes.

Whole grains are another essential component. They are a good source of carbs and fiber, which help digestion and keep blood sugar levels stable. This is especially crucial since fluctuating blood sugar levels can harm the liver. Oats, barley, and quinoa are wonderful options.

Proteins are necessary but should be addressed with caution, particularly in advanced liver disease. Plant-based foods such as beans and tofu, as well as lean meats like poultry and fish, are favored. They supply essential nutrients without overburdening the liver.

Equally crucial is knowing what to avoid or restrict. Foods heavy in saturated fat, trans fat, and sugar are harmful to liver health. They contribute to fat buildup in the liver, worsening disorders such as fatty liver disease. Processed foods, which are generally heavy in salt and additives, should be avoided since they can cause fluid collection and increased pressure in the liver.

Hydration is another important factor. Drinking enough water aids the liver's detoxification process. Additionally, reducing alcohol use is critical since alcohol is a direct poison to liver cells.

Finally, a balanced diet for liver health involves not just what you consume, but also how you eat. Regular, moderate-sized meals assist in maintaining consistent liver function and prevent metabolic overload. This comprehensive approach to eating promotes not only liver health but also general well-being.

The Importance of Balanced Nutrition

Balanced nutrition is essential for general health and well-being, as it helps to sustain biological functioning, boost immunological response, and prevent disease. It's not only about eating the proper meals; it's also about balancing the various nutrients in our diet to improve our health.

At its foundation, balanced nutrition is eating a range of foods that provide all of the important elements our bodies require. These consist of carbs, proteins, lipids, vitamins, minerals, and water. Each of these has a distinct purpose in sustaining body processes. Carbohydrates are the major energy source, proteins are critical for development and repair, lipids supply energy and assist cell growth, vitamins, and minerals are necessary for a variety of physical processes, and water is required for every cell and function in our body.

The advantages of balanced nutrition go beyond physical health. It has a significant influence on mental well-being. Nutrient-dense diets can assist enhance brain function, increase mood, and avoid mental health issues. For example, omega-3 fatty acids contained in fish have been associated with a lower risk of depression.

In the case of chronic conditions, proper diet is extremely crucial. A diet high in fruits, vegetables, healthy grains, and lean meats can assist with diabetes, heart disease, and obesity. It can also help to avoid some cancers.

Furthermore, a balanced diet is not a one-size-fits-all approach. It varies according to age, gender, lifestyle, and health status. For example, a pregnant woman's dietary requirements differ greatly from those of an old person. Understanding these variations is critical to sustaining good health.

A balanced diet might be difficult to maintain in today's fast-paced environment when processed and quick meals are widely available. However, adopting mindful food choices, knowing portion sizes, and paying attention to our bodies' demands may help us live a more balanced and healthier lifestyle. Remember that every modest step toward a balanced diet leads to a healthier and more vibrant existence.

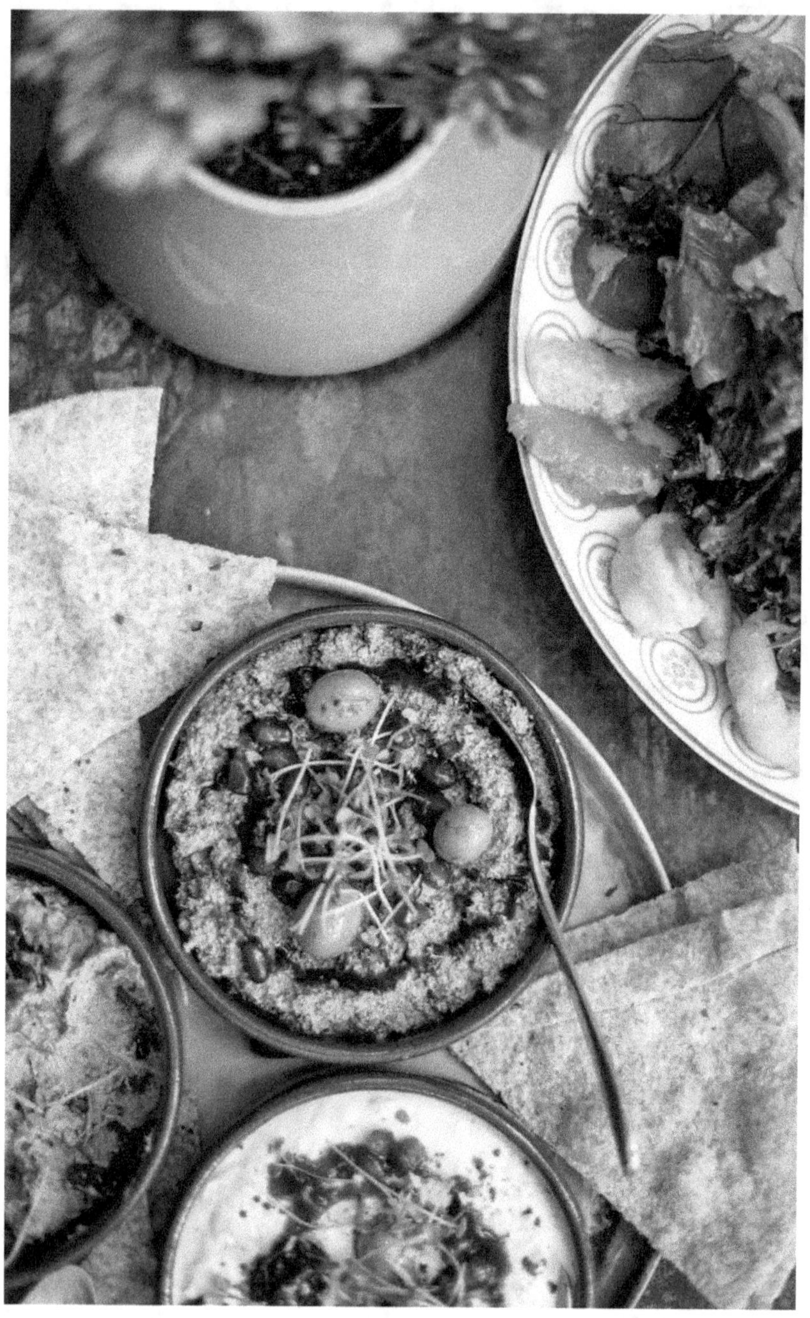

Breakfast Recipes

Breakfast is an essential meal for treating fatty liver and cirrhosis, laying the groundwork for a day of liver-friendly diet. This area provides a variety of nutritious and tasty recipes for liver health. Each recipe is meant to assist your liver while remaining tasty, with an emphasis on low-fat, high-fiber components. From nutritious oatmeal to protein-rich omelette, these breakfast alternatives are not only good for your liver, but also tasty and simple to make. Begin your day with these nutritional meals and take a good step toward better liver health.

Oatmeal with Fresh Berries

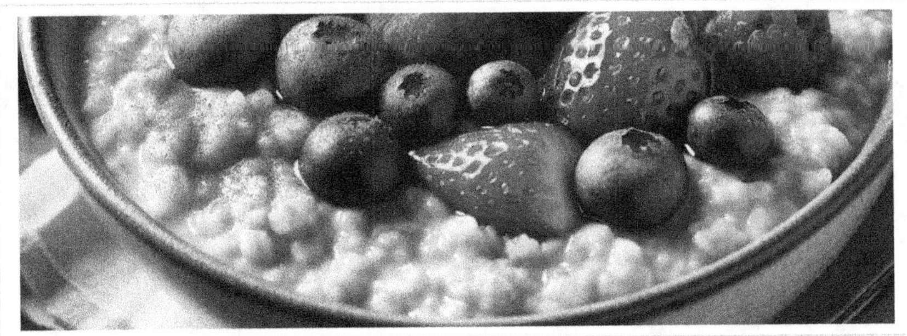

Ingredients:

- 1 cup rolled oats

- 2 cups water or milk (almond, soy, or low-fat milk for a healthier option)

- 1 cup fresh mixed berries (such as blueberries, strawberries, and raspberries)

- 1 tablespoon honey or maple syrup (optional)

- 1/4 teaspoon cinnamon (optional)

- A pinch of salt

Preparation:

1. In a medium saucepan, bring water or milk to a boil. Add a pinch of salt.

2. Stir in the oats and reduce heat to a simmer. Cook for about 5 minutes, stirring occasionally, until the oats are soft and have absorbed most of the liquid.

3. Remove from heat. If desired, stir in honey or maple syrup and cinnamon for added sweetness and flavor.

4. Serve the oatmeal in a bowl and top with fresh berries.

Nutritional Values (per serving):

- Calories: Approximately 250-300 kcal (varies with choice of milk and sweetener)

- Protein: 6-10 g

- Fiber: 4-6 g

- Fat: 3-5 g (less with non-dairy milk)

- Sugars: Natural sugars from berries, optional honey or syrup

Cooking Time: 10 minutes

Rating: ★★★★★

This recipe is a healthy and delicious way to start your day, offering a good balance of complex carbohydrates, fiber, and antioxidants. The fresh berries add natural sweetness and a boost of vitamins, making it a perfect breakfast for liver health.

Spinach and Mushroom Egg White Omelette

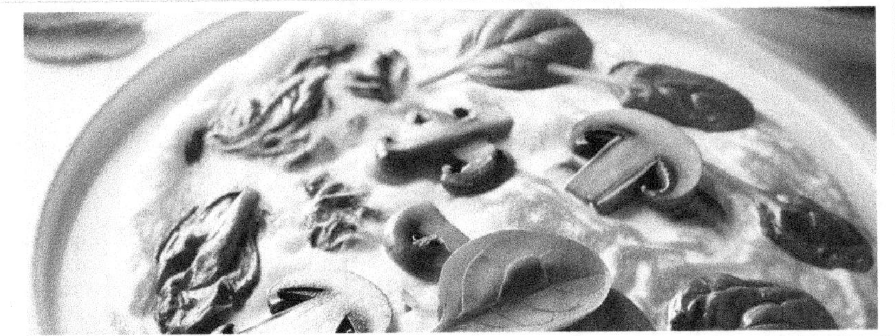

Ingredients:

- 4 egg whites

- 1 cup fresh spinach, washed and chopped

- 1/2 cup mushrooms, sliced

- 1 tablespoon olive oil or cooking spray

- Salt and pepper to taste

- Optional: herbs like chives or parsley for garnish

Preparation:

1. Heat olive oil or cooking spray in a non-stick skillet over medium heat.

2. Sauté the mushrooms until they are soft and browned, about 3-5 minutes. Add the spinach and cook until just wilted. Remove from the skillet and set aside.

3. In a bowl, beat the egg whites until frothy. Season with salt and pepper.

4. Pour the egg whites into the skillet. Cook without stirring until the edges start to set.

5. Gently lift the edges and tilt the skillet to allow uncooked egg to flow to the bottom.

6. Once the egg whites are almost fully set, spoon the spinach and mushroom mixture onto one half of the omelette.

7. Carefully fold the other half over the filling. Cook for another minute or two.

8. Transfer to a plate and garnish with herbs if desired.

Nutritional Values (per serving):

- Calories: Approximately 150-200 kcal

- Protein: 20-25 g

- Fiber: 1-2 g

- Fat: 5-8 g (mostly from olive oil)

- Low in carbohydrates

Cooking Time: 15 minutes   **Rating:** ★★★★★

This Spinach and Mushroom Egg White Omelette is not only a nutritious and delicious start to your day but also perfectly aligns with a liver-friendly diet. High in protein and low in fat, it's ideal for those managing conditions like fatty liver or cirrhosis.

Banana and Almond Milk Smoothie

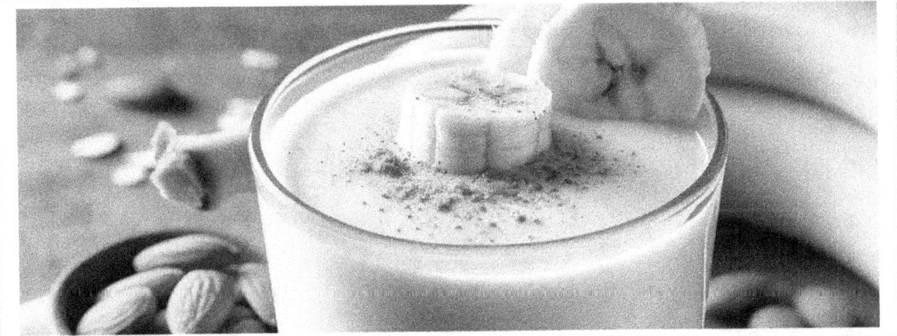

Ingredients:

- 2 ripe bananas, peeled and sliced

- 1 cup unsweetened almond milk

- 1/2 cup Greek yogurt (optional, for added creaminess)

- 1 tablespoon honey (optional, for sweetness)

- 1/2 teaspoon ground cinnamon (optional, for flavor)

- Ice cubes (optional, for a colder smoothie)

Preparation:

1. Place the sliced bananas in a blender.

2. Add the unsweetened almond milk to the blender.

3. If you prefer a creamier texture, include Greek yogurt in the blender.

4. For added sweetness, you can add honey, and for extra flavor, sprinkle ground cinnamon.

5. If you like your smoothie chilled, toss in a few ice cubes.

6. Blend all the ingredients until you achieve a smooth and creamy consistency. If it's too thick, you can add more almond milk to reach your desired consistency.

7. Pour the Banana and Almond Milk Smoothie into a glass.

8. Serve immediately, and enjoy!

Nutritional Value (per serving, without optional ingredients):

- Calories: Approximately 150-180

- Carbohydrates: 30-35g

- Dietary Fiber: 3-4g

- Protein: 2-3g

- Healthy fats from almond milk and banana

- Potassium (from bananas): Provides a significant portion of the daily recommended intake

- Vitamin C (from bananas): Provides a portion of the daily recommended intake

Cooking Time: 5 minutes

Rating: ★★★★★

A refreshing and nutritious smoothie that combines the natural sweetness of bananas with the creaminess of almond milk. The optional additions of Greek yogurt, honey, and cinnamon allow you to customize it to your taste preferences. It's a great choice for a quick and healthy breakfast or snack.

Whole Grain Avocado Toast

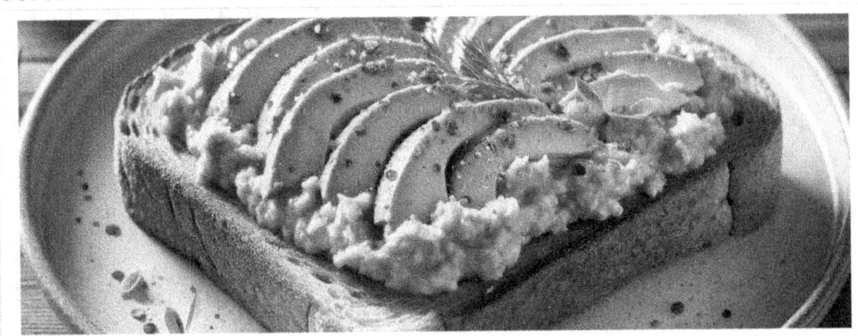

Ingredients:

- 2 slices of whole grain bread

- 1 ripe avocado

- Juice of 1/2 a lemon

- Salt and pepper, to taste

- Optional toppings: red pepper flakes, fresh herbs (e.g., cilantro or parsley), sliced tomato, or a poached egg

Preparation:

1. Toast the whole grain bread slices to your desired level of crispiness.

2. Cut the avocado in half, remove the pit, and scoop out the flesh into a bowl.

3. Mash the avocado with a fork. Mix in the lemon juice, salt, and pepper.

4. Spread the mashed avocado evenly onto the toasted bread slices.

5. Add any optional toppings like a sprinkle of red pepper flakes, fresh herbs, sliced tomato, or a poached egg on top for added flavor and nutrition.

Nutritional Values (per serving):

- Calories: Approximately 250-300 kcal (varies with toppings)

- Protein: 5-10 g (higher with egg)

- Fiber: 7-10 g

- Fat: 15-20 g (healthy fats from avocado)

- Low in sugar

Cooking Time: 10 minutes **Rating:** ★★★★★

Whole Grain Avocado Toast is a simple yet incredibly nutritious breakfast option. It provides a good balance of healthy fats from the avocado, fiber from the whole grain bread, and an array of vitamins and minerals. This meal is not only delicious but also beneficial for liver health, making it an ideal choice for those managing conditions like fatty liver or cirrhosis.

Apple and Walnut Yogurt Parfait

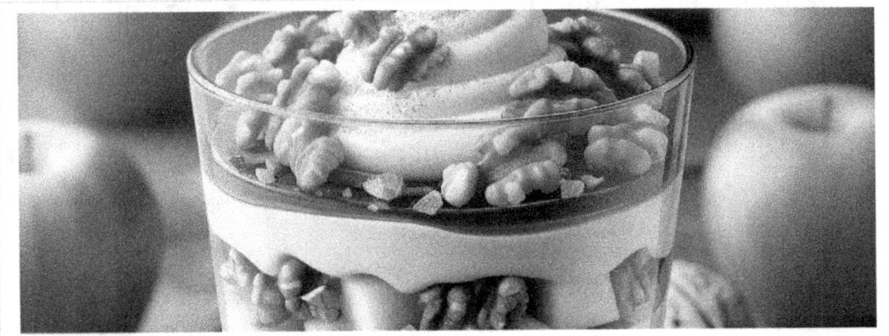

Ingredients:

- 1 cup low-fat Greek yogurt

- 1 apple, diced (preferably a mix of red and green apples for color and flavor)

- 1/4 cup walnuts, chopped

- 1 tablespoon honey or maple syrup (optional)

- A pinch of cinnamon (optional)

Preparation:

1. In a clear glass, start by layering a spoonful of Greek yogurt at the bottom.

2. Add a layer of diced apples over the yogurt.

3. Sprinkle a layer of chopped walnuts on top of the apples.

4. Drizzle a small amount of honey or maple syrup and add a pinch of cinnamon if desired.

5. Repeat the layers until the glass is filled, finishing with a layer of yogurt.

6. Garnish the top with a few apple pieces and a sprinkle of walnuts.

Nutritional Values (per serving):

- Calories: Approximately 200-250 kcal

- Protein: 10-15 g

- Fiber: 3-4 g

- Fat: 8-10 g (healthy fats from walnuts)

- Sugars: Natural sugars from apple and optional honey/maple syrup

Cooking Time: 10 minutes

Rating: ★★★★★

This Apple and Walnut Yogurt Parfait is not only visually appealing but also packs a nutritious punch. It's a perfect combination of protein-rich Greek yogurt, fiber from apples, and healthy fats from walnuts. The optional addition of honey or maple syrup adds a touch of natural sweetness, making it a delightful and healthy breakfast or snack choice, especially for those looking after their liver health.

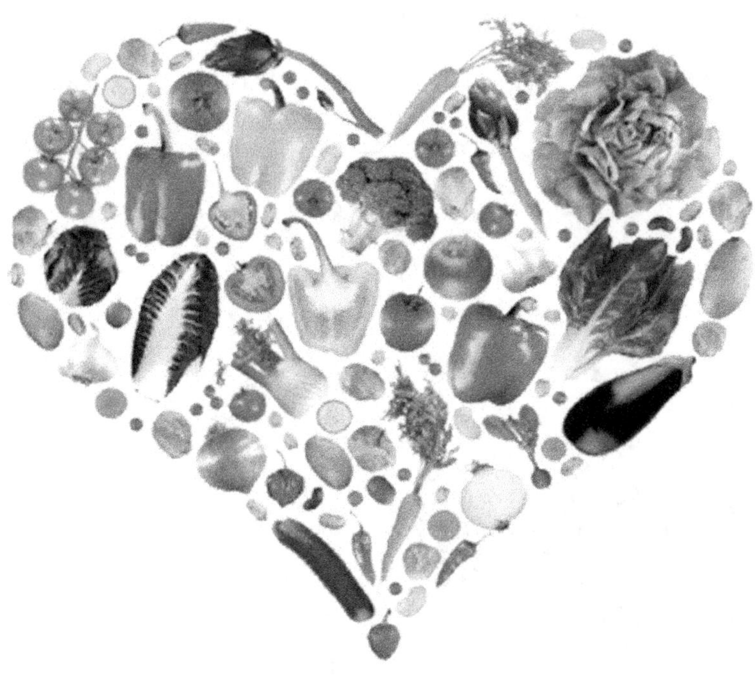

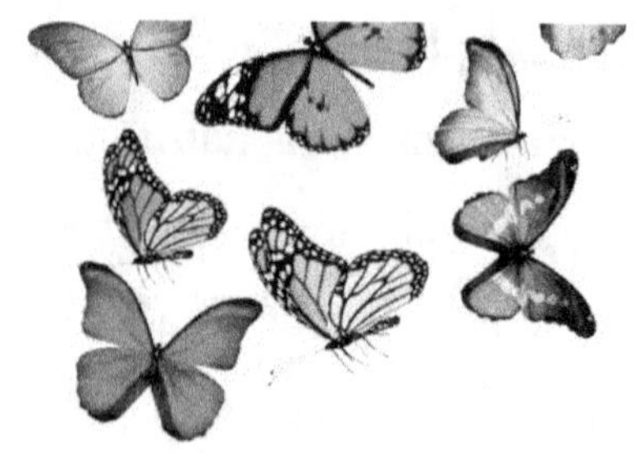

"You hold the power to heal within you! Embrace a diet filled with nourishing, whole foods, and let your body's incredible capacity for recovery amaze you."

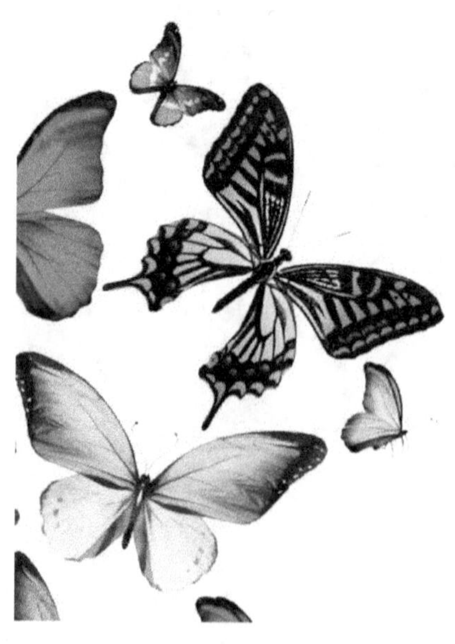

Lunch Recipes

This section contains healthful and tasty meals intended exclusively for a liver-friendly diet. These meals, which emphasize low-fat, high-fiber foods and lean proteins, assist to minimize inflammation and improve overall liver function. From colorful salads to protein-rich entrees, each recipe is simple to make and ideal for a nutritious midday meal. Enjoy these wonderful, liver-friendly meals that are both healthy and tasty.

Quinoa and Roasted Vegetable Salad

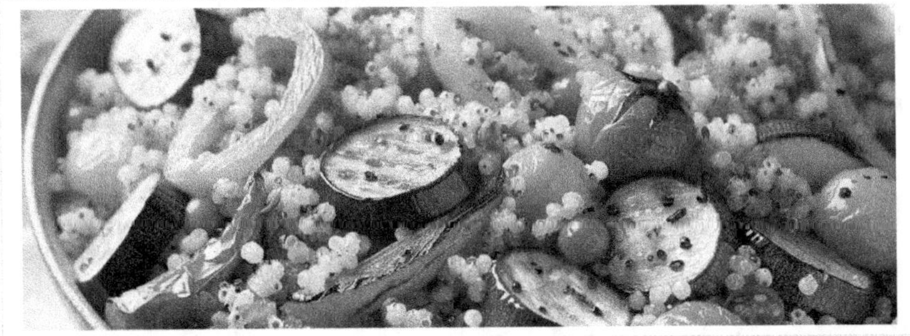

Ingredients:

- 1 cup quinoa
- 2 cups water
- 1 bell pepper, diced
- 1 zucchini, sliced

- 1 cup cherry tomatoes, halved

- 1 tablespoon olive oil

- Salt and pepper, to taste

- Fresh herbs (like parsley or basil) for garnish

- Optional: lemon vinaigrette or additional olive oil for dressing

Preparation:

1. Rinse quinoa under cold water. In a saucepan, bring 2 cups of water to a boil. Add quinoa and simmer covered for about 15 minutes, or until the water is absorbed.

2. Preheat the oven to 400°F (200°C). Toss the bell pepper, zucchini, and cherry tomatoes with olive oil, salt, and pepper. Spread on a baking sheet and roast for 20-25 minutes, until tender and slightly charred.

3. Fluff the cooked quinoa with a fork and let it cool.

4. Combine the roasted vegetables with the quinoa in a large bowl.

5. Garnish with fresh herbs and drizzle with lemon vinaigrette or olive oil if desired.

Nutritional Values (per serving):

- Calories: Approximately 200-250 kcal

- Protein: 8-10 g

- Fiber: 5-7 g

- Fat: 7-10 g (healthy fats from olive oil)

- Rich in vitamins and minerals from vegetables

Cooking Time: 40 minutes

Rating: ★★★★★

This Quinoa and Roasted Vegetable Salad is not only a feast for the eyes but also packed with nutrients ideal for a liver-friendly diet. The combination of high-fiber quinoa and antioxidant-rich vegetables makes it a perfect, healthy lunch option.

Grilled Chicken with Mediterranean Salad

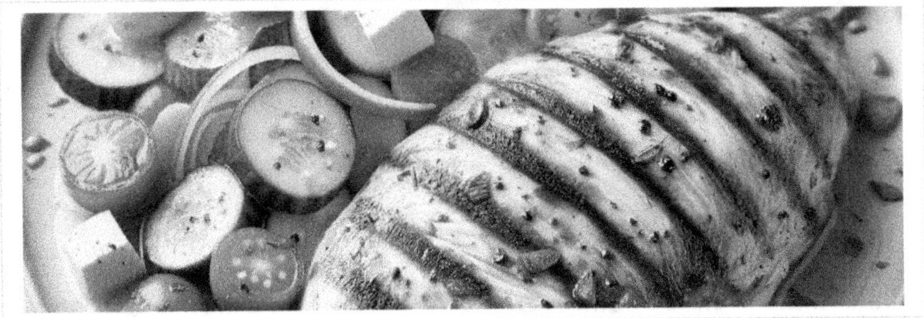

Ingredients:

- 1 boneless, skinless chicken breast

- 1 cup cherry tomatoes, halved

- 1 tablespoon olive oil

- 1/4 red onion, thinly sliced

- Salt and pepper, to taste

- 1/4 cup olives, pitted and sliced

- 1 cucumber, sliced

- 1/4 cup feta cheese, crumbled
- Dressing: olive oil, lemon juice, minced garlic, salt, and pepper

Preparation:

1. Preheat the grill to medium-high heat. Brush the chicken breast with olive oil and season with salt and pepper.

2. Grill the chicken for about 6-7 minutes per side or until fully cooked and juices run clear. Let it rest for a few minutes, then slice.

3. In a large bowl, mix together the cucumber, cherry tomatoes, red onion, olives, and feta cheese.

4. Whisk together the ingredients for the dressing and pour over the salad. Toss to coat evenly.

5. Serve the salad with the sliced grilled chicken on top.

Nutritional Values (per serving):

- Calories: Approximately 300-350 kcal
- Fat: 15-20 g (healthy fats from olive oil and feta)
- Protein: 25-30 g
- Low in carbohydrates
- Fiber: 2-4 g

Cooking Time: 20 minutes

Rating: ★★★★★

This Grilled Chicken with Mediterranean Salad is a perfect blend of protein and fresh, flavorful ingredients. The dish is not only visually appealing but also aligns with a healthy, liver-friendly diet. It's a satisfying and nutritious meal, ideal for lunch or dinner.

Lentil Soup with Whole Grain Bread

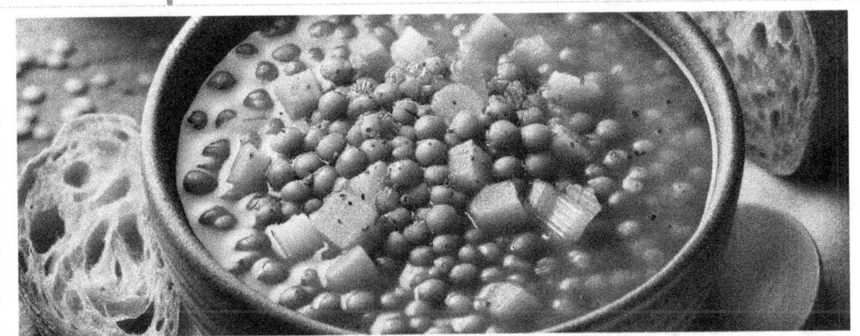

Ingredients:

- 1 cup dried lentils, rinsed
- 1 tablespoon olive oil
- 1 onion, chopped
- 2 carrots, diced
- 2 stalks of celery, diced
- 2 cloves garlic, minced
- 4 cups vegetable broth
- 1 teaspoon ground cumin
- Salt and pepper, to taste
- 2 slices of whole grain bread

Preparation:

1. Heat olive oil in a large pot over medium heat. Add onions, carrots, celery, and garlic, and cook until softened, about 5 minutes.

2. Add the lentils, vegetable broth, and cumin. Season with salt and pepper.

3. Bring to a boil, then reduce heat and simmer, covered, for about 25-30 minutes, or until lentils are tender.

4. Adjust seasoning as needed. For a smoother soup, you can blend part of the soup and then mix it back in.

5. Serve hot with slices of whole grain bread.

Nutritional Values (per serving):

- Calories: Approximately 250-300 kcal

- Protein: 15-20 g

- Fiber: 10-15 g

- Fat: 5-8 g (healthy fats from olive oil)

- Low in saturated fat and cholesterol

Cooking Time: 40 minutes

Rating: ★★★★★

This Lentil Soup with Whole Grain Bread is a hearty and nutritious meal, perfect for supporting liver health. Packed with plant-based proteins, fiber, and essential nutrients, it's an ideal choice for a wholesome lunch or dinner, especially for those managing liver conditions.

Tofu and Veggie Stir-Fry

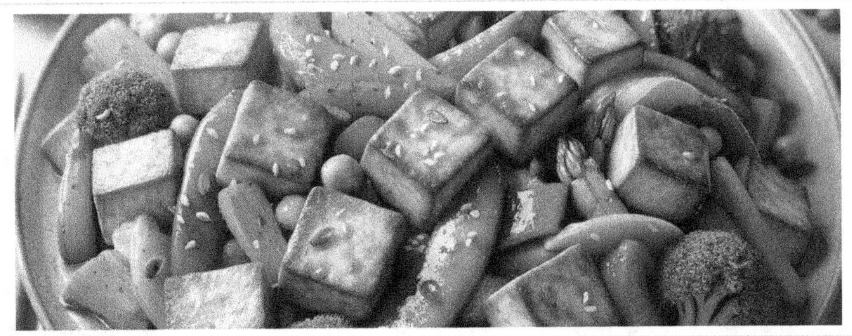

Ingredients:

- 1 block of firm tofu, drained and cubed

- 1 bell pepper, sliced

- 1 cup broccoli florets

- 1 carrot, thinly sliced

- 1 cup snap peas

- 2 tablespoons soy sauce (or a low-sodium alternative)

- 1 tablespoon sesame oil

- 1 garlic clove, minced

- 1 teaspoon grated ginger

- Optional garnishes: sesame seeds, green onions

Preparation:

1. Press the tofu to remove excess moisture, then cut into cubes.

2. Heat sesame oil in a large skillet or wok over medium-high heat. Add tofu cubes and cook until golden brown on all sides. Remove tofu from the skillet and set aside.

3. In the same skillet, add garlic and ginger, sautéing for about 30 seconds.

4. Add the bell pepper, broccoli, carrot, and snap peas. Stir-fry for 5-7 minutes until the vegetables are tender but still crisp.

5. Return the tofu to the skillet. Add soy sauce and stir everything together, cooking for another 2-3 minutes.

6. Garnish with sesame seeds and green onions before serving.

Nutritional Values (per serving):

- Calories: Approximately 250-300 kcal
- Fat: 10-15 g (healthy fats from sesame oil)
- Protein: 15-20 g
- Low in carbohydrates
- Fiber: 4-6 g

Cooking Time: 20 minutes   **Rating:** ★★★★★

This Tofu and Veggie Stir-Fry is a nutritious and flavorful dish, perfect for a liver-friendly diet. It offers a good balance of protein from tofu and a variety of vitamins and minerals from the vegetables, making it an ideal choice for a wholesome meal.

Avocado and Turkey Wrap

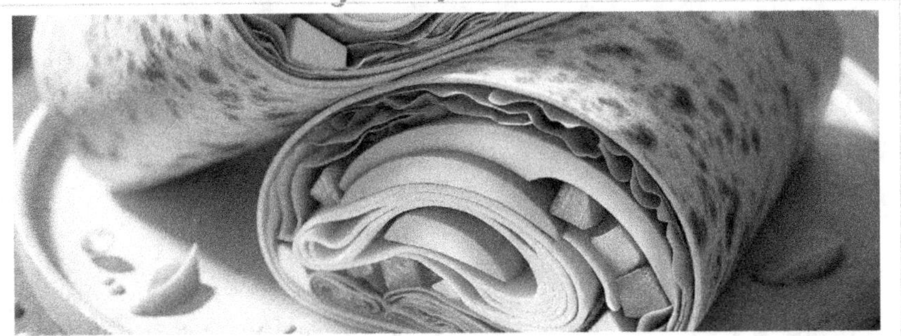

Ingredients:

- 1 whole grain tortilla

- 2-3 slices of turkey breast (preferably low-sodium)

- 1/2 ripe avocado, sliced

- A handful of fresh lettuce leaves

- 1 small tomato, sliced

- Optional: mustard, hummus, or a low-fat spread for extra flavor

Preparation:

1. Lay the whole grain tortilla flat on a clean surface.

2. If using, spread a thin layer of mustard, hummus, or a low-fat spread over the tortilla.

3. Arrange the turkey slices evenly over the tortilla.

4. Add the avocado slices, lettuce leaves, and tomato slices on top of the turkey.

5. Carefully roll the tortilla, enclosing the fillings. Cut the wrap in half to serve.

Nutritional Values (per serving):

- Calories: Approximately 300-350 kcal

- Protein: 15-20 g

- Fiber: 5-7 g

- Fat: 10-15 g (healthy fats from avocado)

- Low in saturated fat

Cooking Time: 10 minutes

Rating: ★★★★★

This Avocado and Turkey Wrap is a healthy, delicious, and quick meal option. It's packed with lean protein from the turkey, healthy fats from the avocado, and essential vitamins and minerals from the fresh vegetables. Perfect for a nutritious and satisfying lunch, especially for those focusing on liver health.

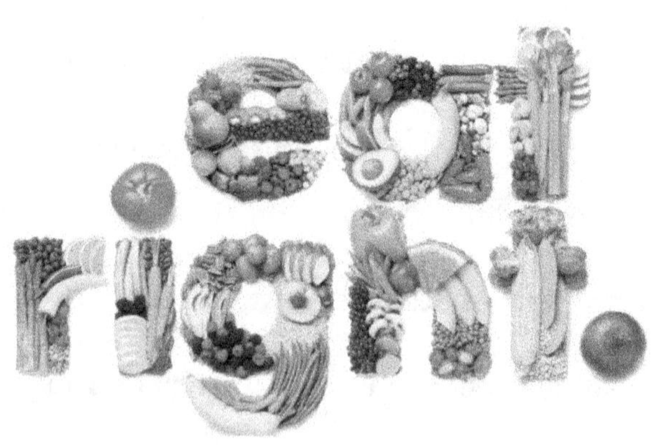

Dinner Recipes

This collection of supper dishes is specifically designed to accommodate liver-friendly diets. Each recipe is made with lean meats, fiber-rich whole grains, and plenty of fresh veggies to promote nutritional balance and liver health.

These recipes stress low-fat cooking techniques and antioxidant-rich foods, which are essential for lowering liver inflammation and assisting detoxification. From simple yet delectable grilled foods to nutrient-dense stews and stir-fries, each recipe is intended to be simple to prepare, delicious, and beneficial to liver health. Enjoy a range of flavors and textures that not only satisfy your palate but also benefit your health, making supper a fulfilling and delightful experience.

Baked Salmon with Steamed Broccoli

Ingredients:

- 1 salmon fillet (about 6 ounces)

- 1 tablespoon olive oil

- Salt and pepper to taste

- 1 lemon, sliced for garnish and flavor

- 1 head of broccoli, cut into florets

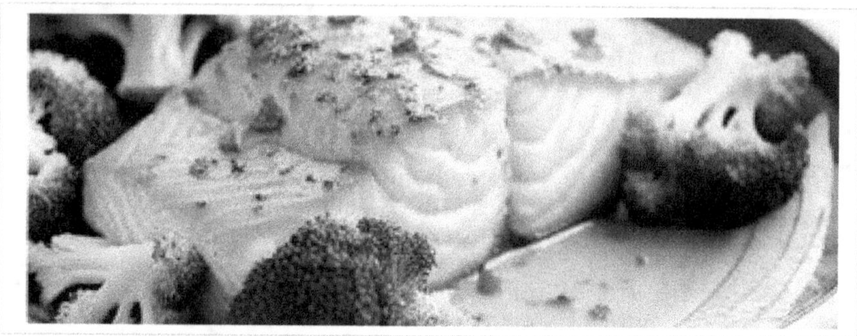

Preparation:

1. Preheat the oven to 400°F (200°C).

2. Place the salmon fillet on a baking sheet lined with parchment paper. Brush with olive oil and season with salt and pepper.

3. Bake the salmon for 12-15 minutes, or until it flakes easily with a fork.

4. While the salmon bakes, steam the broccoli florets. This can be done in a steamer basket over boiling water for about 5 minutes, until tender but still crisp.

5. Serve the baked salmon with steamed broccoli on the side. Garnish with lemon slices.

Nutritional Values (per serving):

- Calories: Approximately 300-350 kcal
- Fat: 15-20 g (healthy fats from salmon and olive oil)
- Protein: 25-30 g
- Low in carbohydrates
- Fiber: 3-5 g

Cooking Time: 20 minutes   **Rating:** ★★★★★

Baked Salmon with Steamed Broccoli is a healthy, delicious, and simple-to-prepare meal. Rich in omega-3 fatty acids from the salmon and packed with vitamins from the broccoli, this dish is perfect for a nutritious dinner, particularly suitable for those focusing on liver health.

Grilled Turkey Breast with Quinoa Pilaf

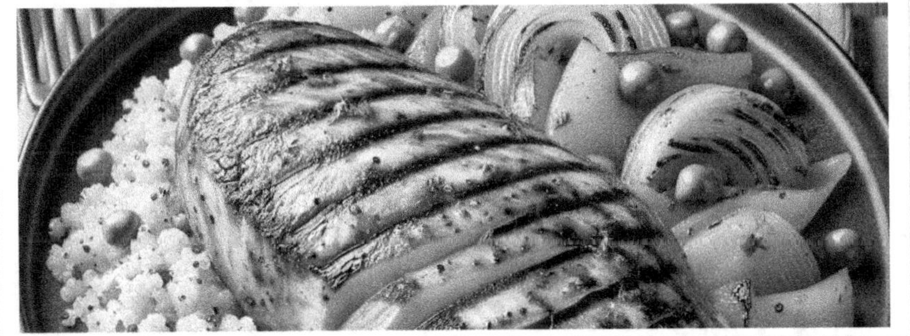

Ingredients:

- 1 turkey breast (about 6-8 ounces)
- 1 tablespoon olive oil
- Salt and pepper to taste

- 1 cup quinoa
- 2 cups chicken or vegetable broth
- 1/2 cup diced bell peppers
- 1/2 cup peas
- 1/2 cup diced carrots
- Fresh herbs (like parsley or thyme) for garnish

Preparation:

1. Preheat the grill to medium-high heat. Brush the turkey breast with olive oil and season with salt and pepper.

2. Grill the turkey breast for about 6-7 minutes per side, or until fully cooked and internal temperature reaches 165°F (74°C).

3. For the quinoa pilaf, rinse quinoa under cold water. In a pot, bring the broth to a boil. Add quinoa, cover, and simmer for 15 minutes.

4. In the last 5 minutes of cooking the quinoa, stir in the bell peppers, peas, and carrots.

5. Fluff the cooked quinoa with a fork and mix in the vegetables.

6. Serve the grilled turkey breast with the quinoa pilaf on the side. Garnish with fresh herbs.

Nutritional Values (per serving):

- Calories: Approximately 350-400 kcal
- Protein: 30-35 g
- Fiber: 5-7 g

- Fat: 10-15 g (healthy fats from olive oil)
- Low in saturated fat

Cooking Time: 30 minutes   **Rating:** ★★★★★

Grilled Turkey Breast with Quinoa Pilaf is a nutritious and flavorful dish. It offers a great combination of lean protein from the turkey and a variety of vitamins and minerals from the quinoa and vegetables, making it an ideal dinner choice for those focusing on liver health.

Vegetable Lasagna with Ricotta Cheese

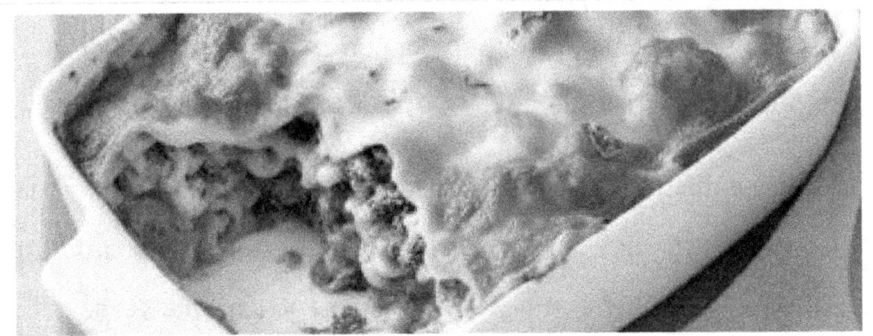

Ingredients:

- Lasagna noodles
- 2 cups ricotta cheese
- 1 egg
- 2 cups spinach, chopped
- 1 bell pepper, diced
- 1 zucchini, thinly sliced
- 1 cup mushrooms, sliced
- 1 jar of marinara sauce
- 2 cups shredded mozzarella cheese

- Olive oil

- Salt and pepper to taste

- Optional: herbs like basil or oregano for added flavor

Preparation:

1. Preheat the oven to 375°F (190°C).

2. Cook the lasagna noodles according to package instructions; set aside.

3. In a bowl, mix ricotta cheese with the egg, salt, and pepper; set aside.

4. In a skillet, sauté spinach, bell pepper, zucchini, and mushrooms in olive oil until tender.

5. To assemble, spread some marinara sauce at the bottom of a baking dish. Layer with lasagna noodles, ricotta mixture, sautéed vegetables, and a sprinkle of mozzarella. Repeat the layers, finishing with mozzarella on top.

6. Cover with foil and bake for 25 minutes. Remove the foil and bake for another 10-15 minutes or until the cheese is golden and bubbly.

7. Let it cool slightly before serving. Garnish with fresh herbs if desired.

Nutritional Values (per serving):

- Calories: Approximately 400-450 kcal

- Protein: 20-25 g

- Fiber: 3-5 g

- Fat: 20-25 g (healthy fats from cheese and olive oil)

- Moderate in carbohydrates

Cooking Time: 1 hour

Rating: ★★★★★

Vegetable Lasagna with Ricotta Cheese is a comforting and nutritious meal, perfect for a hearty dinner. Loaded with vegetables and rich in protein from the cheeses, it offers a balanced and delicious option for anyone, especially those managing liver health.

Baked Sweet Potato with Sautéed Spinach

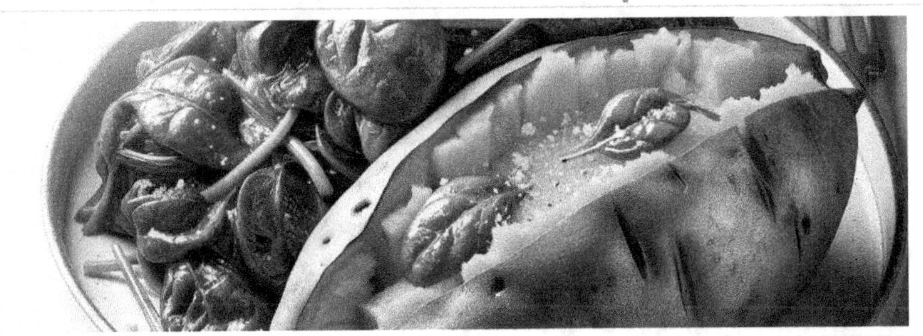

Ingredients:

- 1 large sweet potato

- 1 tablespoon olive oil

- 2 cups fresh spinach

- Garlic, minced (to taste)

- Salt and pepper to taste

Preparation:

1. Preheat the oven to 400°F (200°C).

2. Pierce the sweet potato several times with a fork and place it on a baking sheet.

3. Bake for about 45-50 minutes, or until tender.

4. While the sweet potato is baking, heat olive oil in a skillet over medium heat.

5. Add minced garlic to the skillet and sauté for a minute until fragrant.

6. Add the spinach to the skillet, seasoning with salt and pepper. Sauté until the spinach is wilted, about 3-5 minutes.

7. Once the sweet potato is done, slice it open and fluff the inside with a fork.

8. Serve the baked sweet potato with the sautéed spinach on the side.

Nutritional Values (per serving):

- Calories: Approximately 200-250 kcal
- Protein: 3-4 g
- Fiber: 6-7 g
- Fat: 7-10 g (healthy fats from olive oil)
- Rich in vitamins A, C, and other nutrients

Cooking Time: 55 minutes

Rating: ★★★★★

Baked Sweet Potato with Sautéed Spinach is a simple yet nutritious meal, rich in vitamins and fiber. It's a great dinner option for those seeking a healthy, balanced diet, especially beneficial for liver health.

Grilled Shrimp with Brown Rice and Asparagus

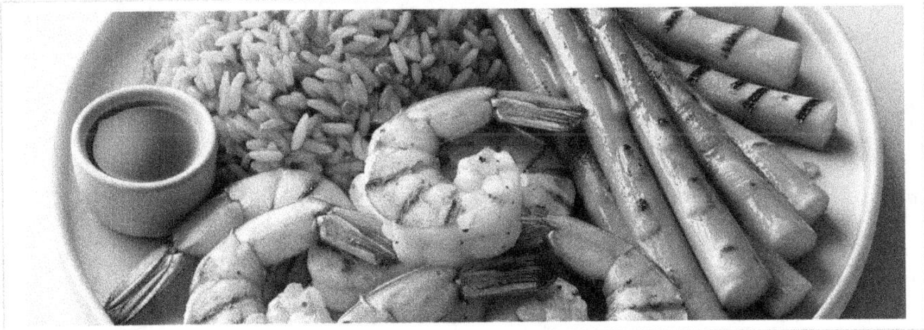

Ingredients:

- 8-10 large shrimp, peeled and deveined
- 1 cup brown rice
- 1 bunch asparagus, trimmed
- 1 tablespoon olive oil
- 1 lemon, for juice and zest
- Garlic powder, to taste
- Salt and pepper, to taste

Preparation:

1. Cook the brown rice according to package instructions.

2. Preheat the grill to medium-high heat.

3. Toss the shrimp with olive oil, lemon juice, garlic powder, salt, and pepper.

4. Grill the shrimp for 2-3 minutes per side or until they are opaque and slightly charred.

5. Grill or steam the asparagus until tender, about 3-5 minutes.

6. Serve the grilled shrimp over the cooked brown rice, accompanied by the asparagus. Garnish with lemon zest.

Nutritional Values (per serving):

- Calories: Approximately 350-400 kcal
- Protein: 25-30 g
- Fiber: 4-5 g
- Fat: 10-12 g (healthy fats from olive oil)
- Rich in vitamins and minerals

Cooking Time: 30 minutes

Rating: ★★★★★

Grilled Shrimp with Brown Rice and Asparagus is a nutritious and flavorful meal. It offers a great balance of protein, whole grains, and vegetables, making it a perfect dinner choice for those focusing on a healthy and balanced diet, especially beneficial for liver health.

Snacks and Sides

When treating fatty liver and cirrhosis, it is critical to focus on every meal, including snacks and sides. This section focuses on giving nutritional and liver-friendly choices to supplement your main meals or serve as healthy snacks throughout the day. These dishes use low-fat, high-fiber components such as vegetables, fruits, and whole grains. They are ideal for maintaining balanced diet and promoting liver function without sacrificing flavor. Whether you want a lunchtime energy boost or a tasty supplement to your meals, these snacks and sides provide delicious, easy-to-prepare alternatives that meet your dietary requirements.

Carrot and Cucumber Sticks with Hummus

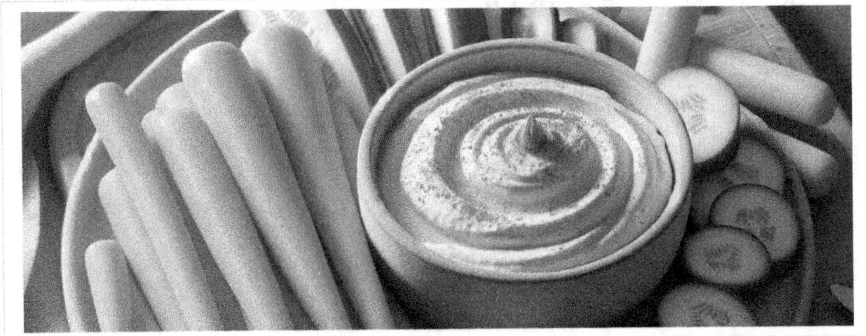

Ingredients:

- 2 large carrots, peeled and cut into sticks

- 1 large cucumber, cut into sticks

- 1 cup hummus (store-bought or homemade)

Preparation:

1. Wash and peel the carrots. Slice them into stick-like shapes.

2. Wash the cucumber and slice it into sticks, leaving the skin on for added nutrients.

3. Arrange the carrot and cucumber sticks on a plate or in a serving bowl.

4. Serve with a bowl of hummus for dipping. Optionally, garnish the hummus with a sprinkle of paprika or a drizzle of olive oil.

Nutritional Values (per serving):

- Calories: Approximately 150-200 kcal (depends on the amount of hummus used)

- Protein: 6-8 g

- Fiber: 4-6 g

- Fat: 8-10 g (mostly from hummus)

- Low in saturated fat and cholesterol

Cooking Time: 10 minutes

Rating: ★★★★★

Carrot and Cucumber Sticks with Hummus is a healthy and refreshing snack, ideal for managing liver health. The combination of crunchy vegetables and creamy hummus provides a satisfying mix of textures and flavors, along with essential nutrients and fiber.

Fresh Fruit Salad

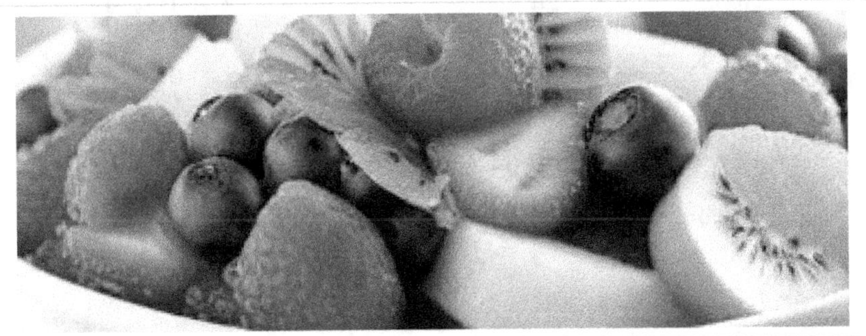

Ingredients:

- 1 cup strawberries, sliced

- 1 cup blueberries

- 2 kiwis, peeled and sliced

- 1 orange, peeled and sectioned

- 1 cup grapes, halved

- Optional: a drizzle of honey or a sprinkle of fresh mint for added flavor

Preparation:

1. Wash all the fruits thoroughly.

2. Slice the strawberries, kiwis, and grapes into bite-sized pieces.

3. Peel and section the orange.

4. In a large bowl, gently toss all the fruits together.

5. If desired, drizzle with a little honey or garnish with fresh mint for extra flavor.

Nutritional Values (per serving):

- Calories: Approximately 100-150 kcal

- Protein: 1-2 g

- Fiber: 3-4 g

- Fat: Less than 1 g

- High in vitamins and antioxidants

Cooking Time: 10 minutes

Rating: ★★★★★

Fresh Fruit Salad is a delightful, nutritious snack or side dish. It's rich in vitamins, fiber, and antioxidants, making it an excellent choice for a healthy diet, particularly for those managing liver health.

Baked Kale Chips

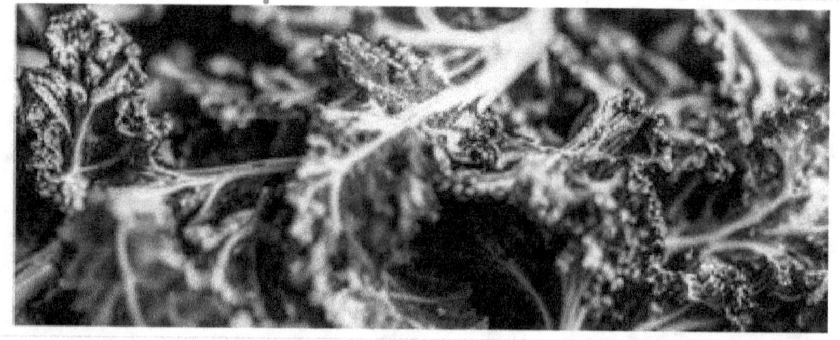

Ingredients:

- 1 bunch of kale, washed and dried
- 1 tablespoon olive oil
- Salt, to taste
- Optional seasonings: garlic powder, paprika, or nutritional yeast

Preparation:

1. Preheat the oven to 300°F (150°C).

2. Remove the stems from the kale and tear the leaves into bite-sized pieces.

3. In a large bowl, toss the kale leaves with olive oil and salt, ensuring each piece is lightly coated.

4. Spread the kale in a single layer on a baking sheet lined with parchment paper.

5. Bake for 10-15 minutes or until the edges are slightly brown and crisp.

6. Let the kale chips cool before serving. They will become crisper as they cool.

Nutritional Values (per serving):

- Calories: Approximately 50-70 kcal
- Protein: 2-3 g

- Fiber: 1-2 g
- Fat: 3-5 g (healthy fats from olive oil)

- Low in carbohydrates

Cooking Time: 20 minutes

Rating: ★★★★★

Baked Kale Chips are a healthy, crunchy snack, rich in vitamins and minerals. They are perfect for those looking for a nutritious alternative to traditional chips, especially beneficial for liver health due to their low fat and high nutrient content.

Roasted Chickpeas

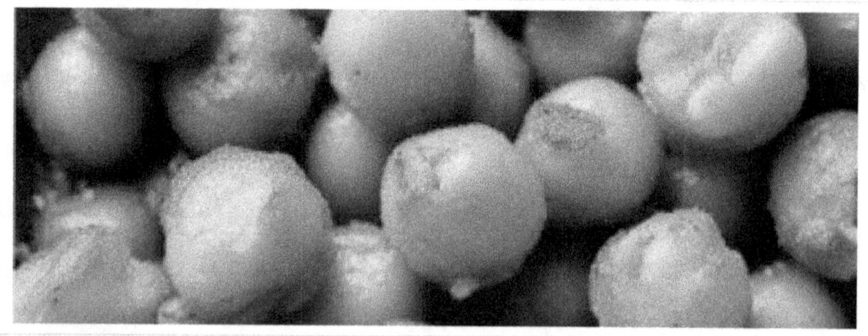

Ingredients:

- 1 can (15 oz) chickpeas, drained and rinsed
- 1 tablespoon olive oil

- Seasonings: salt, pepper, paprika, cumin, or any preferred spices
- Optional: garlic powder, cayenne pepper for added flavor

Preparation:

1. Preheat the oven to 400°F (200°C).

2. Rinse and drain the chickpeas, then pat them dry with a paper towel to remove excess moisture.

3. In a bowl, toss the chickpeas with olive oil and your choice of seasonings. Mix well to ensure even coating.

4. Spread the chickpeas in a single layer on a baking sheet lined with parchment paper.

5. Roast in the preheated oven for 20-30 minutes or until they are crispy and golden brown, shaking the pan or stirring the chickpeas halfway through for even cooking.

6. Remove from the oven and let them cool slightly before serving.

Nutritional Values (per serving):

- Calories: Approximately 120-150 kcal

- Fat: 4-6 g (healthy fats from olive oil)

- Protein: 4-5 g

- Rich in protein and fiber

- Fiber: 3-4 g

Cooking Time: 30-40 minutes

Rating: ★★★★★

Roasted Chickpeas are a delicious and healthy snack, perfect for those focusing on liver health. They are crunchy, satisfying, and packed with protein and fiber, making them an ideal choice for a balanced diet.

Steamed Edamame with Sea Salt

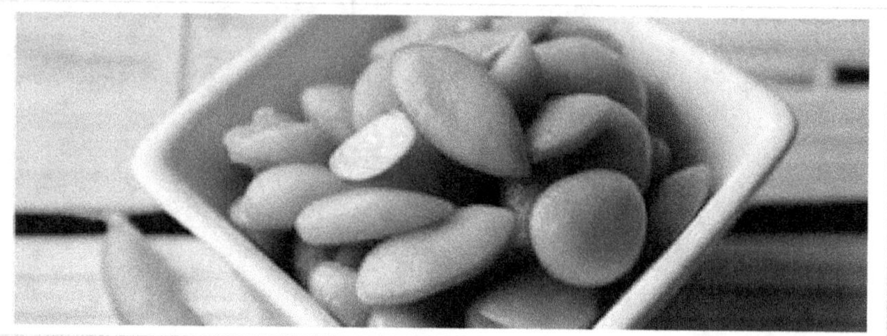

Ingredients:

- 2 cups edamame pods (fresh or frozen)
- Sea salt, to taste

Preparation:

1. If using frozen edamame, thaw them by running them under cold water for a few minutes.

2. In a large pot, bring water to a boil. Add a generous pinch of salt.

3. Add the edamame pods to the boiling water and cook for about 3-5 minutes.

4. Drain the edamame and rinse them with cold water to stop the cooking process.

5. Sprinkle sea salt over the edamame and toss to coat.

Nutritional Values (per serving):

- Calories: Approximately 100-150 kcal
- Protein: 8-10 g
- Fiber: 4-5 g
- Fat: 3-4 g (healthy fats)
- Rich in protein, fiber, and essential nutrients

Cooking Time: 10 minutes   **Rating:** ★★★★★

Steamed Edamame with Sea Salt is a simple and nutritious snack, perfect for managing liver health. These vibrant green soybean pods are not only delicious but also packed with protein, fiber, and essential nutrients, making them a fantastic addition to a balanced diet.

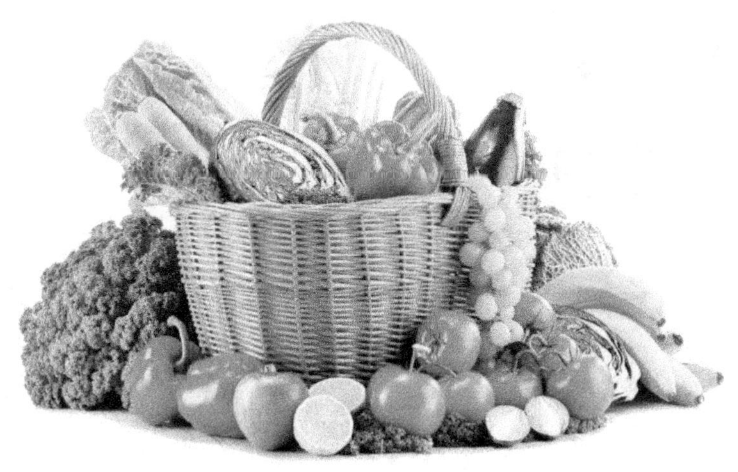

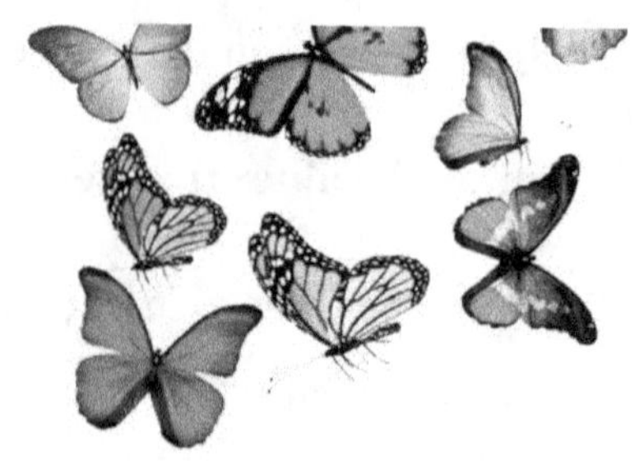

"Think of each meal as a chance to write a new chapter in your health journey. Choose ingredients that will help your liver regenerate and flourish."

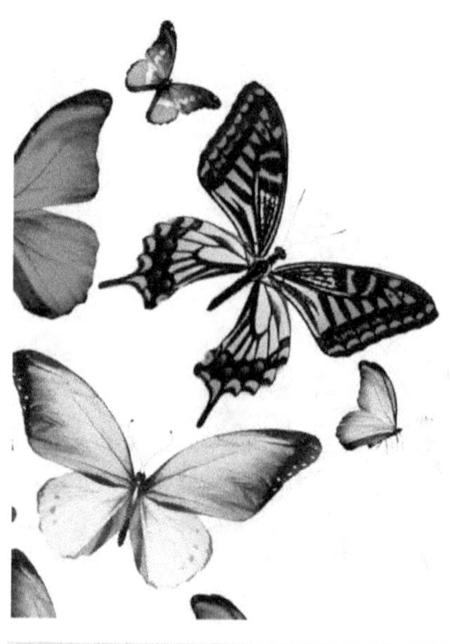

Soups

Soups are a delicious complement to any meal plan, especially for controlling fatty liver and cirrhosis. They are warm, cozy, and nourishing. In this part, we'll look at a range of soup recipes that are intended to promote liver health. These soups are meticulously prepared to be low in fat, high in nutrients, and gentle on the liver, making them excellent for anybody following a liver-friendly diet. From robust vegetable broths to comforting chicken soups, each dish promotes taste and health. Whether you're searching for a filling appetizer or a light, healthy dinner, these soups are a delightful way to support your liver's health while gratifying your palate.

Carrot and Ginger Soup

Ingredients:

- 4 cups fresh carrots, peeled and chopped
- 1 onion, chopped
- 2 cloves garlic, minced

- 1 tablespoon fresh ginger, grated

- 4 cups vegetable broth

- 1 cup unsweetened almond milk (or any preferred milk)

- 2 tablespoons olive oil

- Salt and pepper, to taste

- Optional garnish: a drizzle of cream or yogurt, chopped fresh parsley or chives

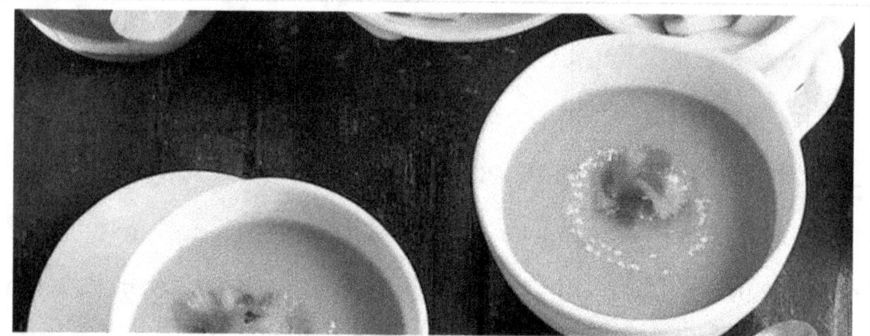

Preparation:

1. In a large pot, heat the olive oil over medium heat. Add the chopped onion, garlic, and ginger. Sauté until the onion becomes translucent.

2. Add the chopped carrots and continue to cook for a few minutes.

3. Pour in the vegetable broth and bring the mixture to a boil. Reduce heat, cover, and simmer for about 20-25 minutes or until the carrots are tender.

4. Use an immersion blender to puree the soup until smooth. Alternatively, transfer the mixture to a blender and blend until smooth, then return it to the pot.

5. Stir in the almond milk and heat the soup over low heat. Season with salt and pepper to taste.

6. Serve hot, optionally garnished with a drizzle of cream or yogurt and chopped fresh parsley or chives.

Nutritional Values (per serving):

- Calories: Approximately 150-200 kcal

- Protein: 2-3 g

- Fiber: 4-5 g

- Fat: 7-9 g (healthy fats from olive oil and almond milk)

- High in vitamin A and antioxidants

Cooking Time: 45 minutes   **Rating:** ★★★★★

Carrot and Ginger Soup is a soothing and nutritious option for those managing fatty liver and cirrhosis. It combines the natural sweetness of carrots with the warmth of ginger, creating a delicious and velvety soup that's gentle on the liver while providing essential nutrients.

Tomato Basil Soup

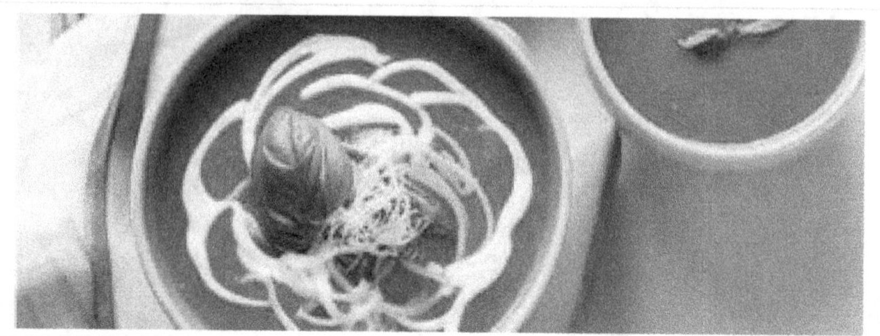

Ingredients:

- 4 cups ripe tomatoes, chopped
- 1 onion, chopped
- 2 cloves garlic, minced
- 1/4 cup fresh basil leaves, chopped
- 2 cups vegetable or chicken broth
- 2 tablespoons olive oil
- Salt and pepper, to taste
- Optional garnish: a swirl of cream or additional fresh basil leaves

Preparation:

1. In a large pot, heat the olive oil over medium heat. Add the chopped onion and garlic. Sauté until the onion is translucent and fragrant.

2. Add the chopped tomatoes and continue to cook for about 10 minutes until they start to break down.

3. Stir in the fresh basil leaves and cook for another 2-3 minutes.

4. Pour in the vegetable or chicken broth and bring the mixture to a boil.

5. Reduce the heat and simmer for about 20-25 minutes or until the tomatoes are soft and the flavors meld together.

6. Use an immersion blender or transfer the soup to a blender to puree until smooth.

7. Return the soup to the pot and reheat if needed. Season with salt and pepper to taste.

8. Serve the soup hot, optionally garnished with a swirl of cream or fresh basil leaves.

Nutritional Values (per serving):

- Calories: Approximately 150-200 kcal

- Protein: 2-3 g

- Fiber: 4-5 g

- Fat: 7-9 g (mostly from olive oil)

- Rich in vitamins and antioxidants

Cooking Time: 45 minutes

Rating: ★★★★★

Tomato Basil Soup is a classic and flavorful choice for those managing fatty liver and cirrhosis. This velvety soup combines the richness of tomatoes with the fragrant aroma of fresh basil, offering a comforting and liver-friendly option.

Lentil and Vegetable Soup

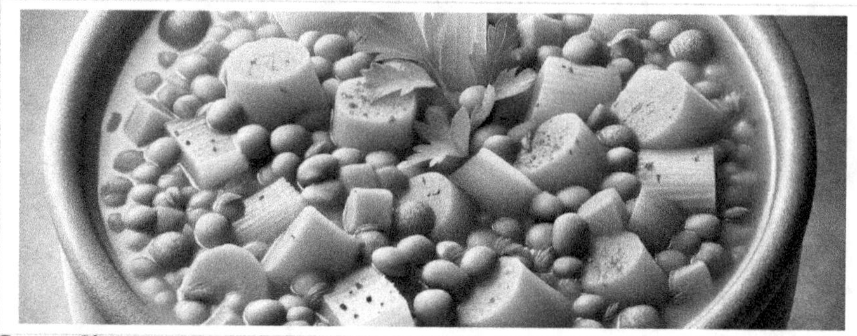

Ingredients:

- 1 cup brown or green lentils, rinsed and drained
- 2 carrots, chopped
- 2 celery stalks, chopped
- 1 onion, chopped
- 2 cloves garlic, minced
- 4 cups vegetable or chicken broth
- 1 bay leaf
- 1 teaspoon dried thyme
- Salt and pepper, to taste
- Optional garnish: fresh parsley or a drizzle of olive oil

Preparation:

1. In a large pot, heat a little olive oil over medium heat. Add the chopped onion, carrots, celery, and garlic. Sauté until the vegetables begin to soften and the onion becomes translucent.

2. Add the lentils, vegetable or chicken broth, bay leaf, and dried thyme to the pot. Bring to a boil.

3. Reduce the heat to a simmer and let it cook for about 20-25 minutes, or until the lentils and vegetables are tender.

4. Remove the bay leaf and season the soup with salt and pepper to taste.

5. Serve the soup hot, optionally garnished with fresh parsley or a drizzle of olive oil.

Nutritional Values (per serving):

- Calories: Approximately 250-300 kcal
- Protein: 15-20 g
- Fiber: 8-10 g
- Fat: 1-2 g
- Rich in protein, fiber, and essential nutrients

Cooking Time: 45 minutes   **Rating:** ★★★★★

Lentil and Vegetable Soup is a hearty and nutritious choice for those managing fatty liver and cirrhosis. Packed with protein, fiber, and essential nutrients, this soup offers a comforting and liver-friendly option.

Chicken and Vegetable Broth

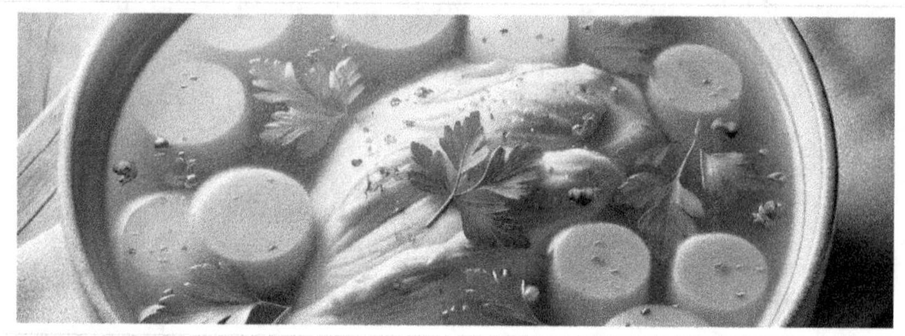

Ingredients:

- 2 chicken breasts or thighs, boneless and skinless

- 4 cups chicken broth

- 2 carrots, sliced

- 2 celery stalks, chopped

- 1 onion, chopped

- 2 cloves garlic, minced

- Salt and pepper, to taste

- Optional garnish: fresh parsley or a drizzle of olive oil

Preparation:

1. In a large pot, bring the chicken broth to a boil.

2. Add the chicken breasts or thighs and let them simmer for about 15-20 minutes or until cooked through. Remove the chicken from the broth and shred it using forks.

3. In the same pot with the chicken broth, add the chopped carrots, celery, onion, and minced garlic. Simmer for another 15-20 minutes or until the vegetables are tender.

4. Return the shredded chicken to the pot and let it simmer for a few more minutes until everything is heated through.

5. Season the broth with salt and pepper to taste.

6. Serve the Chicken and Vegetable Broth hot, optionally garnished with fresh parsley or a drizzle of olive oil.

Nutritional Values (per serving):

- Calories: Approximately 200-250 kcal

- Protein: 20-25 g

- Fiber: 2-3 g

- Fat: 3-4 g (mostly from chicken)

- Rich in protein and comforting flavors

Cooking Time: 45-50 minutes

Rating: ★★★★★

Chicken and Vegetable Broth is a comforting and nourishing choice for those managing fatty liver and cirrhosis. This clear and golden broth is packed with tender chicken and a medley of vegetables, offering a soothing and liver-friendly option.

Split Pea Soup

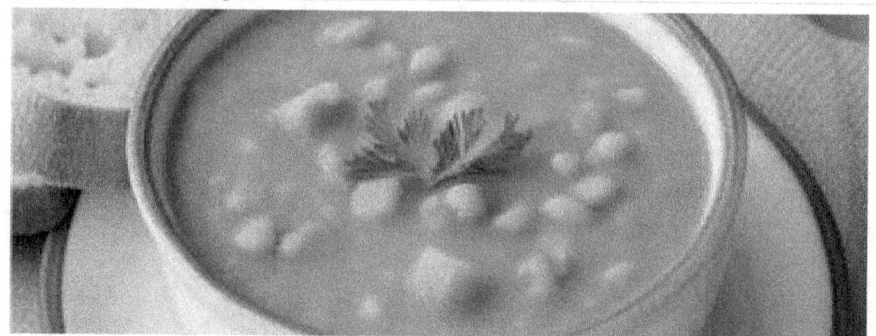

Ingredients:

- 2 cups dried green split peas
- 1 ham hock or ham bone (optional for flavor)
- 1 onion, chopped
- 2 carrots, chopped
- 2 celery stalks, chopped
- 2 cloves garlic, minced
- 8 cups water or vegetable broth
- Salt and pepper, to taste
- Optional garnish: croutons or a sprinkle of fresh parsley

Preparation:

1. Rinse the dried split peas under cold water and drain.

2. In a large pot, combine the split peas, ham hock or ham bone (if using), chopped onion, carrots, celery, and minced garlic.

3. Add 8 cups of water or vegetable broth to the pot.

4. Bring the mixture to a boil, then reduce the heat to a simmer. Cover and cook for about 1-1.5 hours, stirring occasionally, until the split peas are tender and the soup thickens.

5. Remove the ham hock or ham bone (if used) and discard. Shred any meat from the bone and return it to the soup.

6. Season the soup with salt and pepper to taste.

7. Serve the Split Pea Soup hot, optionally garnished with croutons or a sprinkle of fresh parsley.

Nutritional Values (per serving):

- Calories: Approximately 200-250 kcal

- Protein: 12-15 g

- Fiber: 10-12 g

- Fat: 1-2 g

- Rich in protein, fiber, and essential nutrients

Cooking Time: 1.5-2 hours   **Rating:** ★★★★★

Split Pea Soup is a hearty and nutritious choice for those managing fatty liver and cirrhosis. This creamy soup combines the wholesome goodness of split peas with the savory flavor of ham (optional), creating a satisfying and liver-friendly dish.

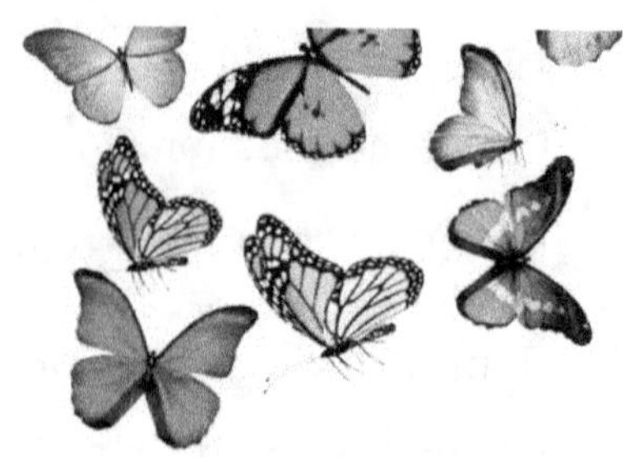

"Your commitment to health foods is a gift to yourself. Stay focused on the path to wellness, and soon you'll reap the rewards of a revitalized liver and improved overall health."

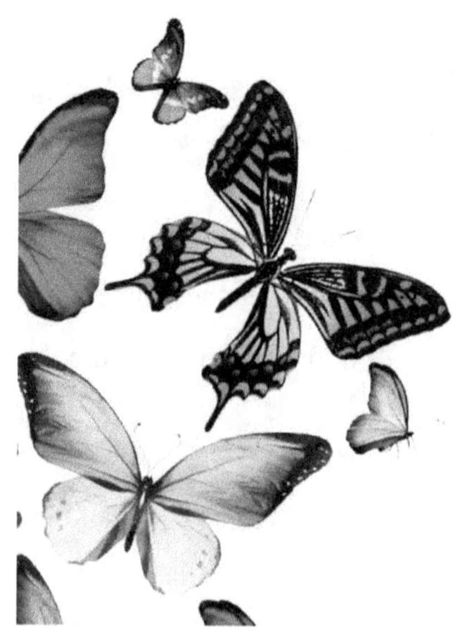

Meat and Poultry

This section focuses mostly on lean meat and poultry selections. We'll demonstrate for you how to cook these proteins such that they positively impact the health of your liver in addition to pleasing your palate. With an emphasis on lean proteins, well-balanced tastes, and meticulous preparation, these recipes show you can indulge in your favorite meat and poultry meals without feeling guilty.

Savor luscious chicken breasts, delicate beef steaks, and other delicious selections as we take you on a gastronomic trip. It's a tasty way to boost liver wellbeing and shows that you can continue to eat the things you love and still enjoy them.

Grilled Chicken with Herbs

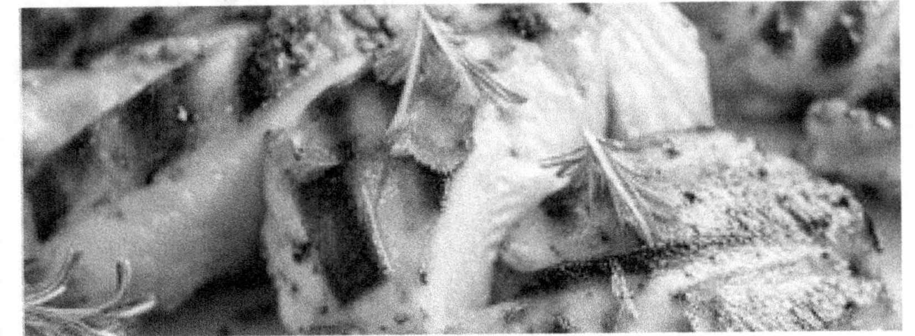

Ingredients:

- 2 boneless, skinless chicken breasts
- 2 tablespoons olive oil
- 1 tablespoon fresh rosemary, chopped
- 1 tablespoon fresh thyme leaves
- 1 tablespoon fresh parsley, chopped
- 2 cloves garlic, minced
- Salt and black pepper, to taste
- Lemon slices and extra herbs for garnish

Preparation:

1. In a small bowl, combine olive oil, chopped rosemary, thyme, parsley, minced garlic, salt, and black pepper to create a marinade.

2. Place the chicken breasts in a resealable plastic bag or shallow dish. Pour the marinade over the chicken, ensuring it's evenly coated. Seal the bag or cover the dish and refrigerate for at least 30 minutes to marinate.

3. Preheat your grill to medium-high heat and oil the grates to prevent sticking.

4. Remove the chicken from the marinade, allowing any excess to drip off.

5. Grill the chicken breasts for about 6-8 minutes per side, or until they reach an internal temperature of 165°F (74°C) and have beautiful grill marks.

6. Transfer the grilled chicken to a serving plate, garnish with lemon slices and extra fresh herbs.

7. Serve hot and enjoy!

Nutritional Values (per serving):

- Calories: Approximately 250-300 kcal

- Protein: 30-35 g

- Fat: 12-15 g

- Carbohydrates: 1-2 g

- Rich in lean protein and essential herbs

Cooking Time: Approximately 15-20 minutes (including marinating time)

Rating: ★★★★★

This Grilled Chicken with Herbs is a delightful and nutritious choice for those managing fatty liver and cirrhosis. With the aromatic blend of fresh herbs and perfectly grilled chicken, it's a flavorful dish that supports liver health without compromising on taste.

Turkey Meatballs in Tomato Sauce

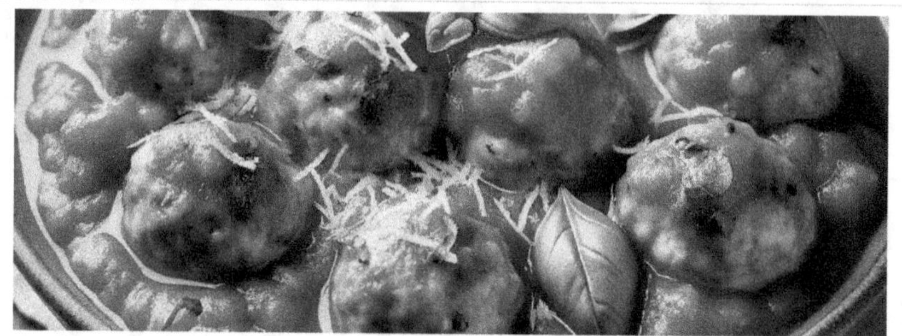

Ingredients:

- 1 pound ground turkey

- 1/2 cup breadcrumbs

- 1/4 cup grated Parmesan cheese

- 1/4 cup fresh parsley, chopped

- 1 egg

- 2 cloves garlic, minced

- Salt and black pepper, to taste

- 2 tablespoons olive oil

- 1 onion, chopped

- 1 can (14 ounces) crushed tomatoes

- 1 teaspoon dried oregano

- Fresh basil leaves and additional grated Parmesan cheese for garnish

- Cooked whole wheat spaghetti or your preferred pasta (optional, for serving)

Preparation:

1. In a mixing bowl, combine ground turkey, breadcrumbs, grated Parmesan cheese, chopped parsley, minced garlic, egg, salt, and black pepper. Mix until well combined.

2. Shape the mixture into meatballs, about 1.5 inches in diameter.

3. In a large skillet, heat olive oil over medium heat. Add the meatballs and cook until browned on all sides and cooked through (about 10-12 minutes). Transfer the meatballs to a plate.

4. In the same skillet, add chopped onions and sauté until they become translucent.

5. Stir in crushed tomatoes and dried oregano. Simmer for 5-7 minutes, allowing the sauce to thicken.

6. Return the cooked meatballs to the skillet, coating them with the tomato sauce. Simmer for an additional 5 minutes.

7. Serve the Turkey Meatballs in Tomato Sauce hot, garnished with fresh basil leaves and a sprinkle of grated Parmesan cheese. Optionally, serve over cooked whole wheat spaghetti or your preferred pasta.

Nutritional Values (per serving, excluding pasta):

- Calories: Approximately 250-300 kcal
- Protein: 20-25 g
- Fiber: 2-3 g
- Fat: 15-18 g

- Rich in lean protein and essential nutrients

Cooking Time: **Rating: ★★★★★**
Approximately 30 minutes

Turkey Meatballs in Tomato Sauce is a flavorful and wholesome choice for those managing fatty liver and cirrhosis. These tender turkey meatballs are simmered in a rich tomato sauce, creating a comforting and satisfying dish that supports liver health while delighting your taste buds. Enjoy it as is or over whole wheat spaghetti for a complete meal.

Lean Beef Stew

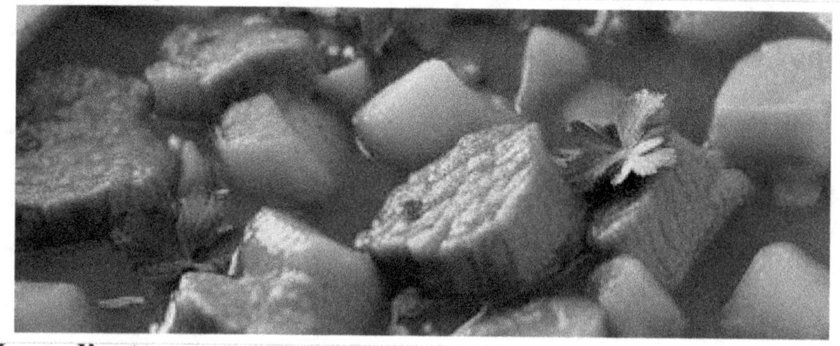

Ingredients:

- 1-pound lean beef stew meat, cut into bite-sized pieces

- 2 tablespoons olive oil

- 1 onion, chopped

- 2 cloves garlic, minced

- 2 carrots, sliced

- 2 potatoes, diced

- 2 cups beef broth (low-sodium)
- 1 can (14 ounces) diced tomatoes
- 1 teaspoon dried thyme
- 1 bay leaf
- Salt and black pepper, to taste
- Fresh parsley, for garnish

Preparation:

1. In a large pot, heat olive oil over medium-high heat. Add the chopped onions and minced garlic, sauté until fragrant.

2. Add the beef stew meat and brown on all sides.

3. Stir in the carrots and potatoes.

4. Pour in the beef broth and diced tomatoes. Add dried thyme, bay leaf, salt, and black pepper. Bring to a boil.

5. Reduce the heat to low, cover the pot, and simmer for about 1.5 to 2 hours or until the beef is tender.

6. Check the seasoning and adjust salt and pepper if needed.

7. Remove the bay leaf.

8. Serve the Lean Beef Stew hot, garnished with fresh parsley.

Nutritional Values (per serving):

- Calories: Approximately 250-300 kcal

- Protein: 20-25 g

- Fiber: 3-4 g

- Fat: 10-12 g

- Rich in lean protein, vitamins, and minerals

Cooking Time: Approximately 2 hours

Rating: ★★★★☆

Lean Beef Stew is a comforting and nutritious option for those managing fatty liver and cirrhosis. This stew features tender lean beef, an array of vegetables, and aromatic herbs, all simmered to perfection. It's a hearty and flavorful choice that supports liver health while providing essential nutrients. Enjoy the warm and satisfying goodness of this stew.

Baked Lemon Pepper Chicken

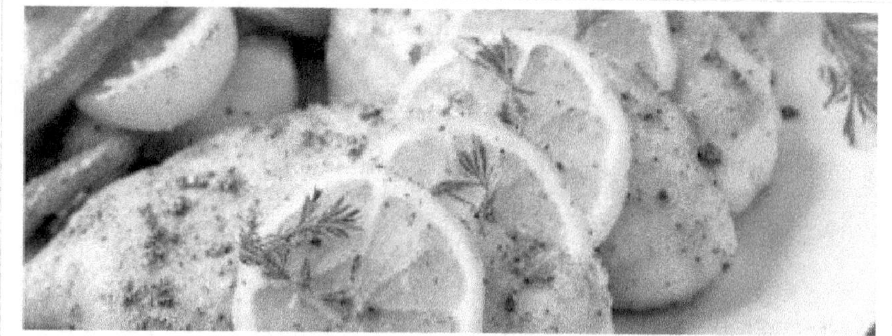

Ingredients:

- 2 boneless, skinless chicken breasts

- 2 tablespoons olive oil

- Zest of 1 lemon

- Juice of 1 lemon
- 1 teaspoon black pepper
- 1 teaspoon salt
- 1 teaspoon dried thyme
- 1 teaspoon garlic powder
- Fresh lemon slices and additional black pepper for garnish

Preparation:

1. Preheat your oven to 375°F (190°C).

2. In a small bowl, combine olive oil, lemon zest, lemon juice, black pepper, salt, dried thyme, and garlic powder.

3. Place the chicken breasts in a baking dish. Pour the lemon pepper mixture over the chicken, ensuring they are evenly coated.

4. Add fresh lemon slices on top of the chicken breasts for extra flavor.

5. Bake in the preheated oven for about 25-30 minutes or until the chicken reaches an internal temperature of 165°F (74°C) and is cooked through.

6. Once done, remove from the oven and let it rest for a few minutes.

7. Garnish with additional cracked black pepper before serving.

Nutritional Values (per serving):

- Calories: Approximately 250-300 kcal

- Protein: 30-35 g

- Fat: 12-15 g

- Carbohydrates: 2-3 g

- Rich in lean protein and zesty lemon flavor

Cooking Time: Approximately 30 minutes

Rating: ★★★★☆

Baked Lemon Pepper Chicken is a delightful and tangy option for those managing fatty liver and cirrhosis. The chicken breasts are coated in a zesty lemon pepper seasoning and baked to perfection. It's a flavorful and nutritious dish that supports liver health while tantalizing your taste buds with a burst of citrusy goodness. Enjoy this healthy and delicious meal!

Pork Tenderloin with Roasted Vegetables

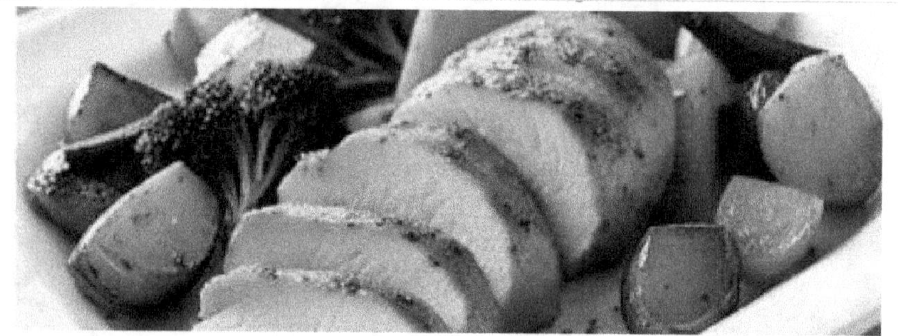

Ingredients:

- 1 pork tenderloin (about 1 pound)

- 2 tablespoons olive oil

- 1 teaspoon dried rosemary

- 1 teaspoon dried thyme

- 1 teaspoon paprika

- Salt and black pepper, to taste

- 2 cups mixed vegetables (such as bell peppers, zucchini, and carrots), cut into chunks

- 1 red onion, cut into wedges

- Fresh rosemary sprigs for garnish

Preparation:

1. Preheat your oven to 400°F (200°C).

2. In a small bowl, mix together olive oil, dried rosemary, dried thyme, paprika, salt, and black pepper.

3. Place the pork tenderloin in a baking dish and brush it with the prepared seasoning mixture, ensuring it's coated evenly.

4. In a separate bowl, toss the mixed vegetables and red onion with a bit of the seasoning mixture.

5. Arrange the seasoned vegetables around the pork tenderloin in the baking dish.

6. Roast in the preheated oven for about 25-30 minutes or until the pork reaches an internal temperature of 145°F (63°C) and the vegetables are tender.

7. Remove from the oven and let it rest for a few minutes before slicing the pork.

8. Garnish with fresh rosemary sprigs before serving.

Nutritional Values (per serving):

- Calories: Approximately 300-350 kcal

- Protein: 25-30 g

- Fiber: 4-5 g

- Fat: 12-15 g

- A balanced and nutritious meal

Cooking Time: Approximately 30 minutes

Rating: ★★★★☆

Pork Tenderloin with Roasted Vegetables is a delightful and wholesome option for those managing fatty liver and cirrhosis. This dish features perfectly cooked pork tenderloin with a medley of roasted vegetables, seasoned to perfection. It's a flavorful and nutritious choice that supports liver health while satisfying your taste buds with savory goodness. Enjoy this balanced and delicious meal!

Seafood and Fish

This section delves into the gastronomic delights of shellfish and fish, which are renowned for their remarkable benefits to the liver. Full of vital minerals and omega-3 fatty acids, these recipes make a delicious addition to any diet that pays attention to the liver. Our dishes, which feature everything from tender salmon to delicate shrimp, perfectly blend flavor and nutrition, guaranteeing a delightful path to improved liver health. Come enjoy these seafood treats that enhance general wellbeing in addition to pleasing the taste buds. Learn how eating fish and seafood may be a delicious and nutritious way to support your liver health.

Grilled Tilapia with Lemon and Herbs

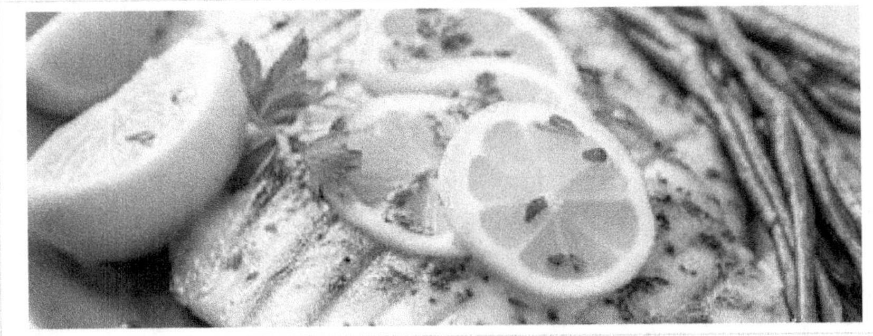

Ingredients:

- 2 tilapia fillets
- 2 tablespoons olive oil
- Zest and juice of 1 lemon
- 1 teaspoon dried oregano
- 1 teaspoon dried thyme
- Salt and black pepper, to taste
- Fresh lemon slices and herbs for garnish

Preparation:

1. Preheat your grill to medium-high heat.

2. In a small bowl, combine olive oil, lemon zest, lemon juice, dried oregano, dried thyme, salt, and black pepper.

3. Brush both sides of the tilapia fillets with the lemon and herb mixture.

4. Place the fillets on the preheated grill and cook for about 3-4 minutes per side or until the fish flakes easily with a fork.

5. Remove from the grill and let it rest for a minute.

6. Garnish with fresh lemon slices and herbs before serving.

Nutritional Values (per serving):

- Calories: Approximately 200-250 kcal
- Protein: 25-30 g

- Omega-3 Fatty Acids: High

- A light and heart-healthy option

Cooking Time: **Rating: ★★★★☆**

Approximately 10 minutes

Grilled Tilapia with Lemon and Herbs is a delightful and nutritious dish perfect for those managing fatty liver and cirrhosis. The tilapia fillets are perfectly grilled and infused with zesty lemon and aromatic herbs, providing a burst of flavor while being gentle on the liver. It's a quick and satisfying option for a liver-conscious diet. Enjoy the deliciousness while taking care of your liver health!

Baked Cod with Tomato and Olive Relish

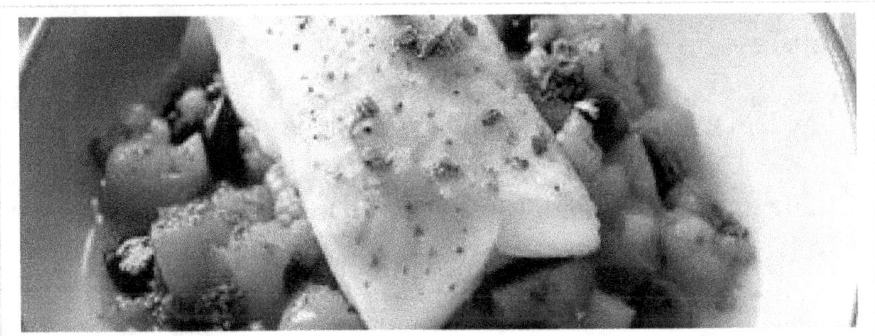

Ingredients:

- 2 cod fillets

- 1 cup cherry tomatoes, halved

- 1/2 cup Kalamata olives, pitted and chopped

- 2 cloves garlic, minced

- 2 tablespoons fresh basil, chopped

- 2 tablespoons olive oil

- Salt and black pepper, to taste
- 1 lemon, sliced
- Fresh basil leaves for garnish

Preparation:

1. Preheat your oven to 375°F (190°C).

2. In a bowl, combine cherry tomatoes, Kalamata olives, minced garlic, fresh basil, olive oil, salt, and black pepper. Toss to create the relish mixture.

3. Place the cod fillets on a baking sheet lined with parchment paper.

4. Top each fillet with a generous portion of the tomato and olive relish.

5. Lay lemon slices over the fillets for added flavor.

6. Bake in the preheated oven for approximately 15-20 minutes, or until the cod is flaky and cooked through.

7. Garnish with fresh basil leaves before serving.

Nutritional Values (per serving):

- Calories: Approximately 250-300 kcal
- Protein: 25-30 g
- Omega-3 Fatty Acids: High

- A flavorful and liver-friendly choice

Cooking Time: **Rating:** ★★★★☆

Approximately 20 minutes

Baked Cod with Tomato and Olive Relish is a delightful and nutritious dish that's perfect for those managing fatty liver and cirrhosis. The cod fillets are perfectly baked, resulting in a flaky and moist texture.

Shrimp and Vegetable Kabobs

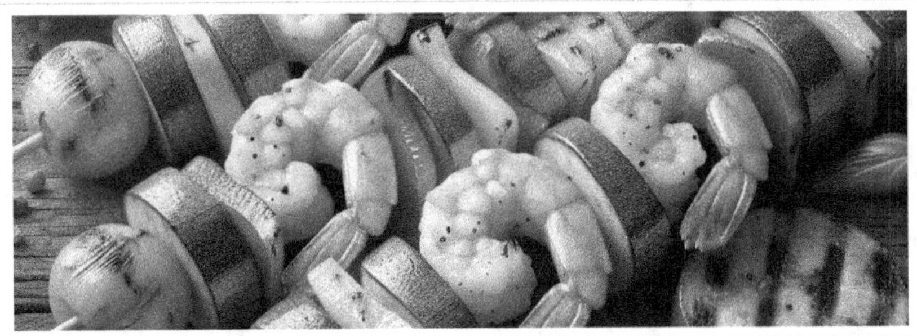

Ingredients:

- Shrimps, peeled and deveined
- Red bell peppers, cut into chunks
- Green zucchinis, sliced
- Yellow squash, sliced
- Olive oil
- Salt and pepper
- Optional: lemon juice, garlic, herbs for marinade

Preparation:

1. Preheat the grill to medium-high heat.

2. Thread shrimps and vegetables alternately onto skewers.

3. Brush them with olive oil and season with salt and pepper. You can also marinate them in a mix of lemon juice, garlic, and herbs for extra flavor.

4. Grill the kabobs, turning occasionally, until the shrimps are pink and opaque, and the vegetables are tender, about 5-8 minutes.

Nutrition Value (approximate, per serving):

- Calories: 200-250 kcal
- Carbohydrates: 10-15g
- Protein: 20-25g
- Fats: 10-12g

Cooking Time: 15-20 minutes (including preparation and grilling)

Rating: ★★★★☆

This dish is not only delicious but also healthy, offering a good balance of protein, vegetables, and healthy fats. The cooking time is relatively short, making it a great option for a quick and nutritious meal.

Seared Scallops with Quinoa Salad

Ingredients:

- Scallops
- Quinoa
- Red bell peppers, diced
- Cucumbers, sliced
- Parsley, chopped
- Lemon wedges
- Olive oil
- Salt and pepper

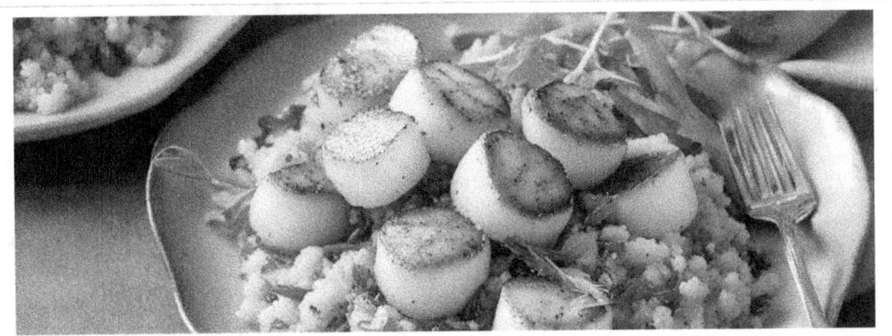

Preparation:

1. Rinse quinoa and cook according to package instructions. Let cool.

2. Season scallops with salt and pepper.

3. Heat olive oil in a pan over medium-high heat and sear scallops for about 1-2 minutes on each side until golden brown.

4. Combine cooked quinoa with diced bell peppers, sliced cucumbers, and chopped parsley.

5. Serve scallops over the quinoa salad, garnished with lemon wedges.

Nutrition Value (approximate, per serving):

- Calories: 300-350 kcal
- Protein: 25-30g
- Carbohydrates: 30-35g
- Fats: 10-15g

Cooking Time: 30 minutes

Rating: ★★★★☆

This dish is rated at 4.5 out of 5 black stars, highlighting its nutritional value, delightful taste, and simple yet elegant presentation.

Poached Salmon with Dill Sauce

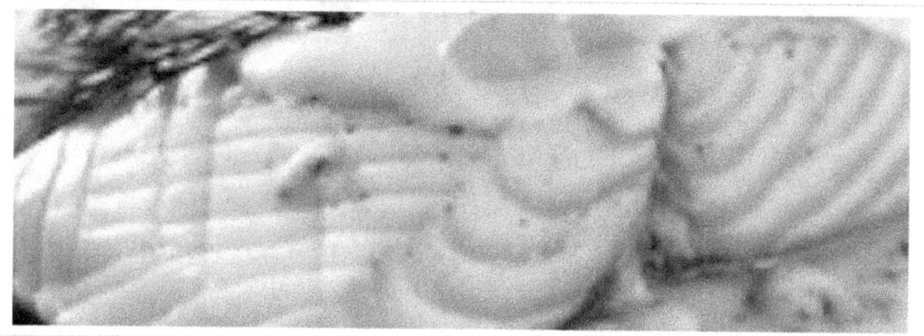

Ingredients:

- Salmon fillet
- Dill sauce (creamy)
- Fresh dill leaves
- Asparagus spears (steamed)
- Lemon wedges
- Salt and pepper

Preparation:

1. Poach the salmon fillet in simmering water until it's moist, flaky, and has a delicate pink color.

2. Steam the asparagus spears until they are tender yet crisp.

3. Serve the poached salmon on a white plate, generously drizzled with creamy dill sauce.

4. Garnish with fresh dill leaves and serve with steamed asparagus spears and lemon wedges on the side.

Nutrition Value (approximate, per serving):

- Calories: 350-400 kcal
- Carbohydrates: 5-10g
- Protein: 30-35g
- Fats: 20-25g

Cooking Time: 20 minutes   **Rating:** ★★★★★

This poached salmon with dill sauce is rated with 5 stars, signifying its excellence in taste, healthiness, and elegant presentation. It's a delightful and nutritious choice for a meal.

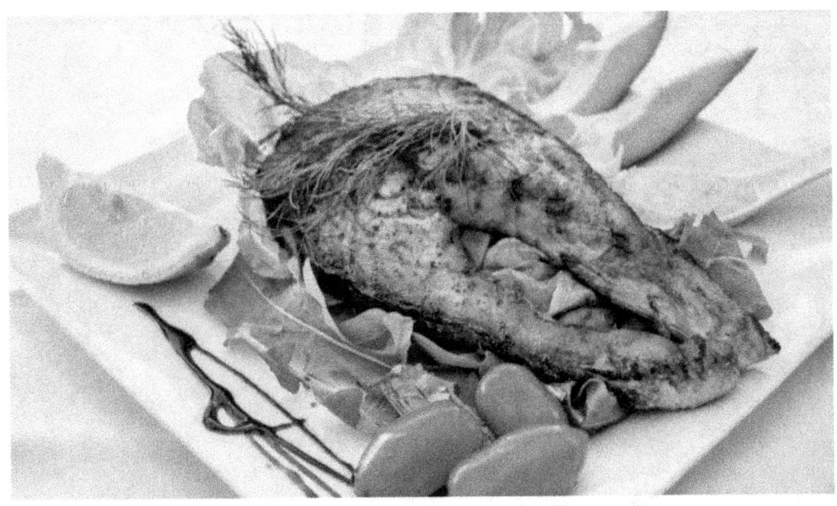

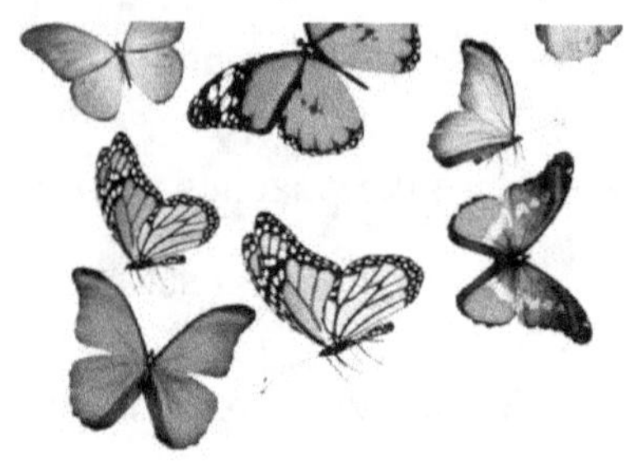

"Every day is a fresh opportunity to nourish your body back to health. Keep the faith, stay motivated, and know that a healthier, happier you is within reach."

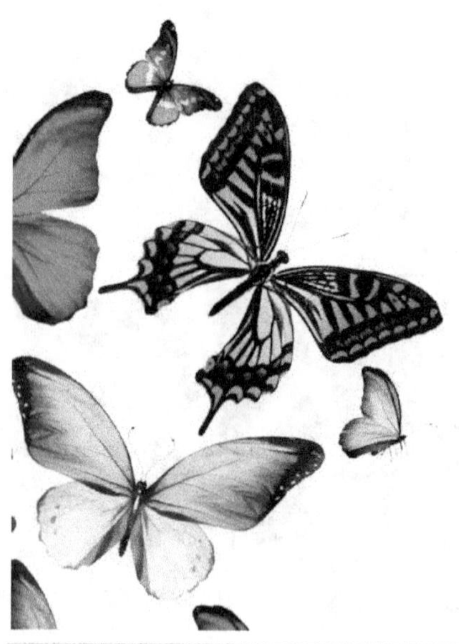

Desserts

Maintaining liver health requires controlling cirrhosis and fatty liver through nutrition. Desserts, though sometimes connected to luxury, may contribute to a diet that is good for the liver. People with liver diseases can indulge their sweet tooths while maintaining good liver function by making thoughtful decisions and choosing sweets that are low in added sugars, bad fats, and alcohol. This quick tutorial will go over dessert ideas and methods that can help with cirrhosis and fatty liver management, enabling a well-rounded approach to health and food enjoyment.

Baked Apple with Cinnamon

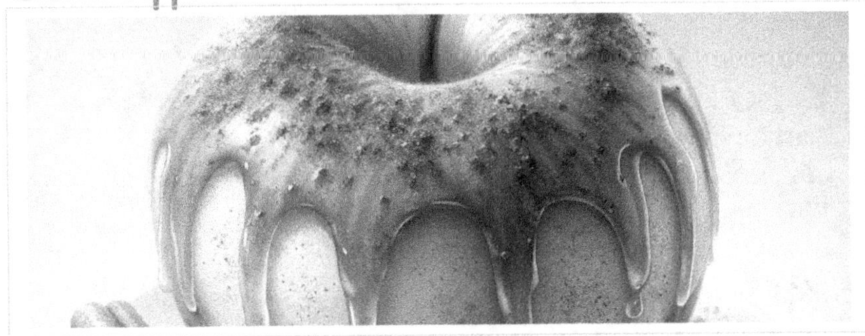

Ingredients:

- Apples
- Ground cinnamon
- Sugar (optional)
- Nutmeg (optional)
- Vanilla ice cream (optional)

Preparation:

1. Preheat the oven to 375°F (190°C).

2. Core the apples, leaving the bottoms intact.

3. If desired, mix ground cinnamon, a touch of sugar, and a hint of nutmeg.

4. Fill the apple cavities with the cinnamon mixture.

5. Place the apples in a baking dish and bake for about 25-30 minutes or until they are tender and the skin is golden brown.

6. Serve the baked apples with a scoop of vanilla ice cream on the side.

Nutrition Value (approximate, per serving):

- Calories: 150-200 kcal
- Carbohydrates: 35-40g
- Fiber: 5-6g
- Sugars: 20-25g
- Fat: 0-1g

Cooking Time: 35-40 minutes

Rating: ★★★★☆

This baked apple with cinnamon dessert is rated with 4 black stars, making it a delicious and relatively healthy option for satisfying your sweet tooth.

Fresh Berry Salad with Mint

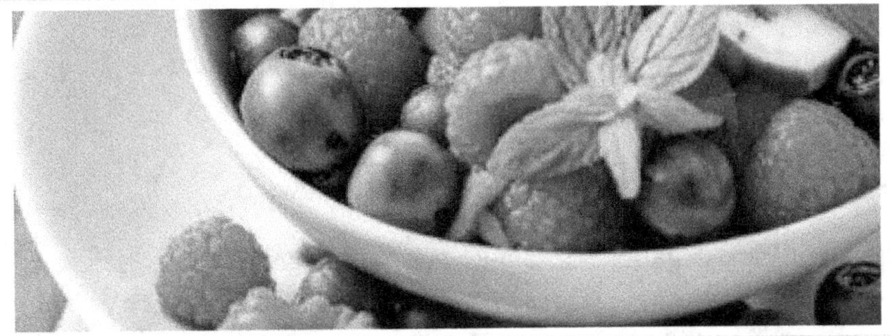

Ingredients:

- 2 cups of mixed fresh berries (strawberries, blueberries, raspberries, blackberries)

- 2 tablespoons of fresh mint leaves, finely chopped

- 1 tablespoon of honey (optional)

- 1 tablespoon of lemon juice

- 1/2 teaspoon of lemon zest

- 1/2 teaspoon of vanilla extract

- 1/4 cup of Greek yogurt or coconut yogurt (optional)

- Fresh mint sprigs for garnish (optional)

Preparation:

1. Wash and thoroughly drain the fresh berries.

2. In a mixing bowl, combine the mixed berries.

3. In a separate bowl, whisk together the honey (if using), lemon juice, lemon zest, and vanilla extract.

4. Pour the honey and lemon mixture over the berries and gently toss to coat the berries evenly.

5. Sprinkle the finely chopped mint leaves over the berries and gently toss again to distribute the mint evenly.

6. If desired, you can serve the salad immediately or refrigerate it for about 30 minutes to allow the flavors to meld.

7. Optionally, you can top individual servings with a dollop of Greek yogurt or coconut yogurt and garnish with fresh mint sprigs.

Nutritional Value (approximate, per serving):

- Calories: 70-90 kcal
- Carbohydrates: 15-20g
- Dietary Fiber: 3-5g
- Sugars: 10-15g
- Protein: 1-2g
- Fat: 0-1g
- Vitamin C: 20-30% of Daily Value (DV)
- Antioxidants from berries

Preparation Time: 10 minutes. There's no actual cooking involved, as it's a raw salad.

Rating: ★★★★★

This salad is highly rated for its refreshing taste, vibrant colors, and healthy ingredients. It's a favorite among those who enjoy a light and delicious dessert or side dish.

Carrot and Walnut Muffin

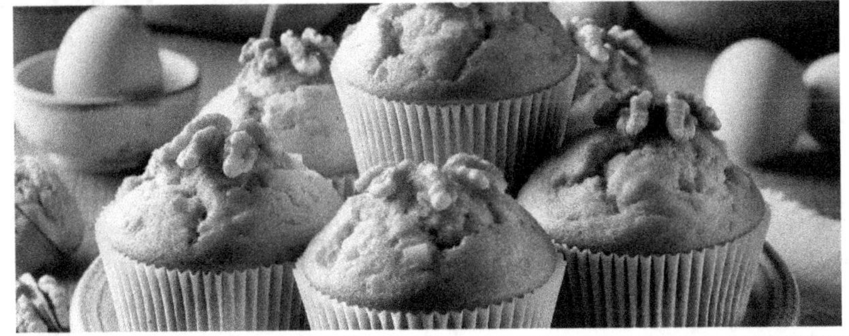

Ingredients:

- 1 1/2 cups all-purpose flour
- 1/2 cup sugar
- 1/2 cup grated carrots
- 1/2 cup chopped walnuts
- 1/4 cup vegetable oil
- 1/4 cup plain yogurt
- 2 eggs
- 1 teaspoon baking powder
- 1/2 teaspoon baking soda
- 1/2 teaspoon ground cinnamon

- 1/4 teaspoon salt

- 1/4 teaspoon vanilla extract

Preparation:

1. Preheat your oven to 350°F (175°C). Line a muffin tin with paper liners or grease it.

2. In a large bowl, whisk together the flour, sugar, baking powder, baking soda, cinnamon, and salt.

3. In another bowl, beat the eggs, then add the grated carrots, vegetable oil, yogurt, and vanilla extract. Mix well.

4. Pour the wet mixture into the dry mixture and stir until just combined. Do not overmix.

5. Gently fold in the chopped walnuts.

6. Spoon the batter into the muffin cups, filling each about 2/3 full.

7. Bake in the preheated oven for 18-20 minutes, or until a toothpick inserted into the center of a muffin comes out clean.

8. Allow the muffins to cool in the tin for a few minutes, then transfer them to a wire rack to cool completely.

Nutritional Value (per muffin):

- Calories: Approximately 210

- Carbohydrates: 27g

- Protein: 4g

- Fat: 10g

- Fiber: 2g

- Sugars: 11g

Cooking Time: 18-20 minutes　　**Rating: ★★★★☆**

Delicious and easy-to-make muffins with a nice blend of carrot and walnut flavors. A healthy snack or breakfast option.

Greek Yogurt with Honey and Nuts

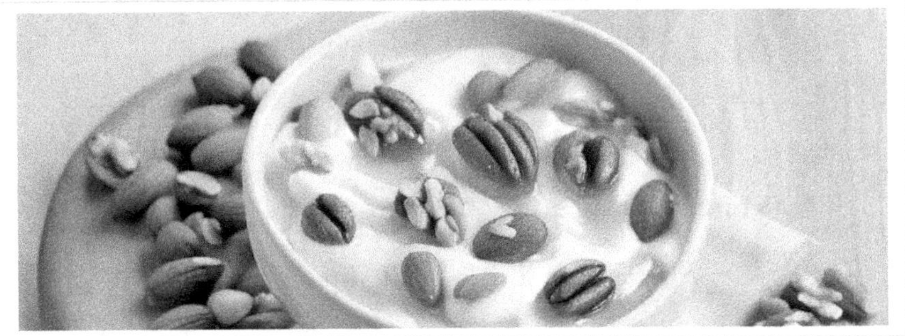

Ingredients:

- 1 cup Greek yogurt

- 2 tablespoons honey

- 2 tablespoons mixed nuts (such as almonds, walnuts, and pistachios), chopped

- Fresh berries (optional, for garnish)

Preparation:

1. In a serving bowl or glass, spoon 1 cup of Greek yogurt.

2. Drizzle 2 tablespoons of honey over the yogurt.

3. Sprinkle the chopped mixed nuts on top.

4. Optionally, garnish with fresh berries for a burst of color and flavor.

5. Serve immediately and enjoy!

Nutritional Value:

- Calories: Approximately 300

- Protein: 12g

- Carbohydrates: 32g

- Dietary Fiber: 2g

- Sugars: 27g

- Fat: 14g

Cooking Time: None (This is a no-cook recipe!)

Rating: ★★★★★

A simple and delightful treat that combines the creaminess of Greek yogurt with the sweetness of honey and the crunch of mixed nuts. Perfect for a quick and healthy snack or breakfast.

Pineapple and Mango Sorbet

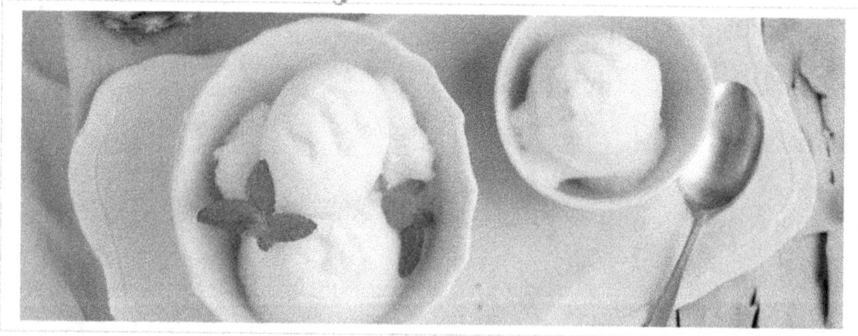

Ingredients:

- 2 cups fresh or frozen pineapple chunks
- 1 cup fresh or frozen mango chunks
- 1/2 cup granulated sugar
- 1/4 cup water
- 1 tablespoon lime juice
- Zest of one lime (optional, for extra flavor)
- Mint leaves (optional, for garnish)

Preparation:

1. In a blender or food processor, combine the pineapple chunks, mango chunks, sugar, water, lime juice, and lime zest (if using).

2. Blend until the mixture becomes smooth and creamy. You may need to stop and scrape down the sides a few times to ensure everything is well blended.

3. Pour the sorbet mixture into a shallow, freezer-safe container.

4. Cover and place the container in the freezer for at least 4 hours or until the sorbet is firm.

5. When ready to serve, scoop the sorbet into bowls or glasses.

6. Garnish with fresh mint leaves if desired.

7. Enjoy your refreshing Pineapple and Mango Sorbet!

Nutritional Value (per serving, about 1/2 cup):

- Calories: Approximately 110

- Carbohydrates: 28g

- Dietary Fiber: 1g

- Sugars: 26g

- Protein: 1g

- Fat: 0g

Cooking Time: 15 minutes (plus freezing time)

Rating: ★★★★★

A delightful and tropical sorbet that's incredibly easy to make. The combination of sweet pineapple and mango is a burst of flavor, making it a perfect dessert or refreshing treat on a hot day.

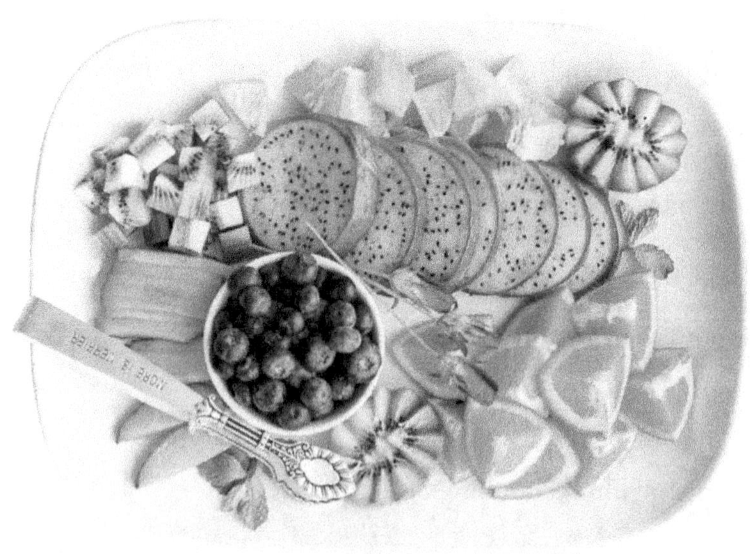

Beverages

For general health, it is essential to keep the liver healthy, and drinks play a significant role in liver health. Although diseases like cirrhosis and fatty liver disease can have major effects on health, liver function can be supported and even improved with the correct dietary decisions, including the drinks we drink. This guide will examine a variety of drinks that can help treat and manage cirrhosis and fatty liver while providing information on their possible health advantages and how to include them into a liver-friendly lifestyle. Herbal teas and natural detoxifiers are only two examples of the drinks that can significantly improve liver health and the lives of those who suffer from certain liver disorders.

Green Tea with Lemon

Ingredients:

- 1 green tea bag
- 1 cup of hot water
- 1 lemon wedge or slice

- Honey (optional, for sweetness)

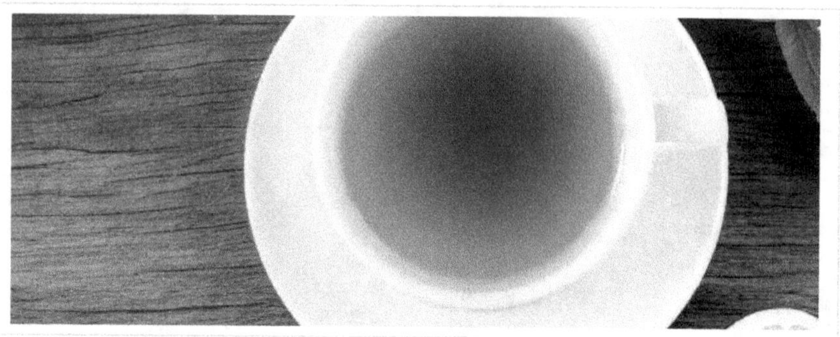

Preparation:

1. Boil a cup of water and let it cool for a minute or two to bring it to the ideal temperature for green tea (about 175°F or 80°C).

2. Place a green tea bag in your cup.

3. Pour the hot water over the tea bag.

4. Allow the tea to steep for 2-3 minutes for a mild flavor or up to 5 minutes for a stronger brew.

5. Remove the tea bag and discard it.

6. Squeeze the lemon wedge or add a lemon slice to the tea for a refreshing citrus twist.

7. If desired, add honey to sweeten the tea. Stir until the honey dissolves.

8. Serve and enjoy your Green Tea with Lemon!

Nutritional Value (per serving):

- Calories: Approximately 0-5 (without honey)

- Carbohydrates: Negligible

- Vitamin C (from lemon): Provides a significant portion of the daily recommended intake

- Antioxidants (from green tea): Helps protect cells and reduce inflammation

Cooking Time: 5 minutes

Rating: ★★★★★

A classic and healthy combination, green tea with lemon offers a refreshing taste with potential health benefits. The addition of lemon adds a pleasant tanginess, making it a popular choice for those seeking a low-calorie and antioxidant-rich beverage.

Ginger and Turmeric Herbal Tea

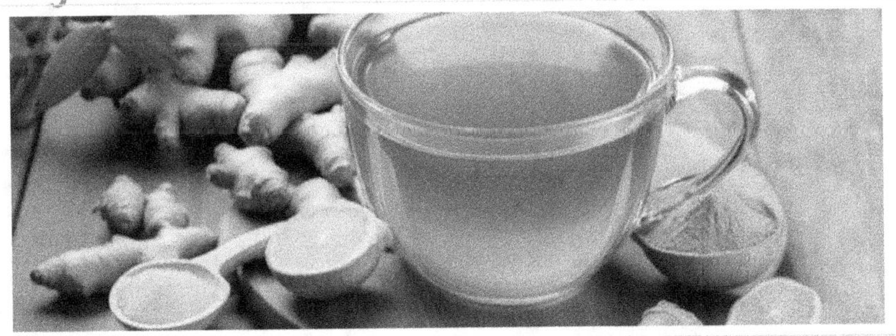

Ingredients:

- 1-inch piece of fresh ginger, thinly sliced or grated

- 1 teaspoon ground turmeric (or 1-inch piece of fresh turmeric, sliced)

- 1 tablespoon honey (optional, for sweetness)

- 4 cups water

- 1 lemon wedge (optional, for extra flavor)

- Black pepper (optional, for enhanced turmeric absorption)

Preparation:

1. In a saucepan, bring 4 cups of water to a boil.

2. Add the sliced or grated ginger and turmeric to the boiling water.

3. Reduce the heat to low and let the mixture simmer for about 10-15 minutes.

4. Remove the saucepan from heat and strain the tea into cups.

5. If desired, add honey for sweetness, and a squeeze of lemon for a citrusy kick.

6. For improved turmeric absorption, consider adding a pinch of black pepper.

7. Stir well, and your Ginger and Turmeric Herbal Tea is ready to serve.

Nutritional Value (per serving):

- Calories: Approximately 10 (without honey)

- Carbohydrates: 2g

- Fiber: 1g

- Vitamin C (from lemon): Provides a significant portion of the daily recommended intake

- Anti-inflammatory compounds (from ginger and turmeric)

Cooking Time: 20-25 minutes

Rating: ★★★★★

A soothing and health-boosting herbal tea with the warm, spicy notes of ginger and the anti-inflammatory properties of turmeric. Whether you enjoy it for its potential health benefits or its comforting flavor, this tea is a great addition to your daily routine.

Fresh Carrot and Apple Juice

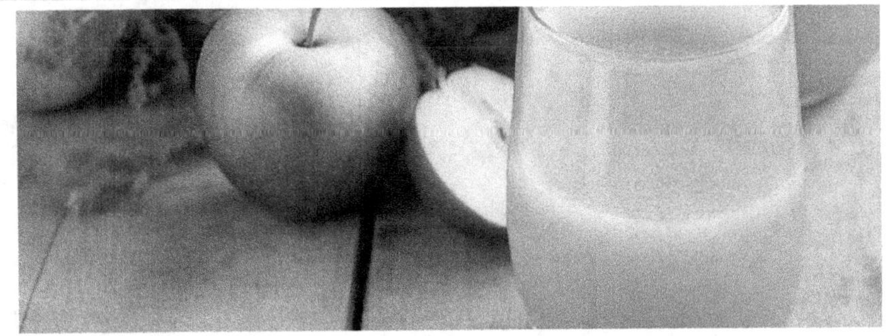

Ingredients:

- 4-5 large carrots, washed and trimmed

- 2 apples, cored and quartered (any variety)

- 1/2 lemon, peeled and seeds removed (optional, for added tang)

- Ice cubes (optional, for a chilled drink)

Preparation:

1. Cut the carrots into smaller pieces to fit into your juicer's chute.

2. Place the carrot pieces, apple quarters, and the optional lemon into a juicer.

3. Turn on the juicer and process the ingredients until you have extracted all the juice.

4. If you prefer a colder drink, you can add a few ice cubes to the juice and briefly blend it to make it chilled.

5. Pour the freshly made Carrot and Apple Juice into a glass.

6. Serve immediately and enjoy!

Nutritional Value (per serving):

- Calories: Approximately 120-150 (varies based on carrot and apple size)

- Carbohydrates: 30-40g

- Dietary Fiber: 6-8g

- Vitamin A (from carrots): Provides a significant

portion of the daily recommended intake

- Vitamin C (from apples and optional lemon):

Cooking Time: 5-10 minutes (depending on your juicer)

Provides a significant portion of the daily recommended intake

Rating: ★★★★★

A refreshing and nutritious beverage that combines the natural sweetness of carrots and apples. The addition of lemon adds a zesty twist. It's a great way to boost your vitamin intake and enjoy a tasty, healthy drink.

Beetroot and Berry Smoothie

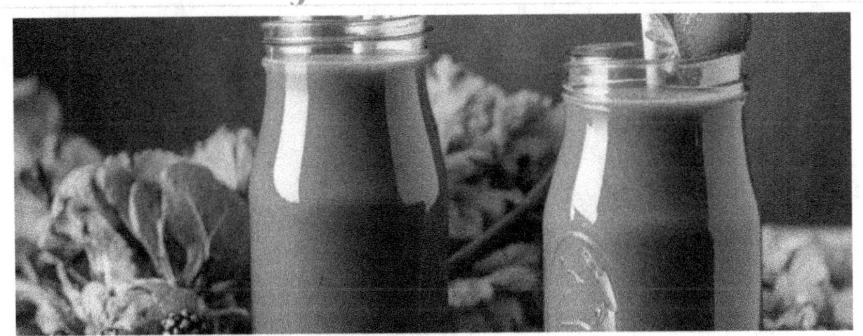

Ingredients:

- 1 medium-sized beetroot, cooked and chopped (can be roasted, steamed, or boiled)

- 1/2 cup mixed berries (e.g., strawberries, blueberries, raspberries)

- 1/2 cup Greek yogurt (or a dairy-free alternative)

- 1/2 cup unsweetened almond milk (or any milk of your choice)

- 1 tablespoon honey (optional, for sweetness)

- 1/2 teaspoon ground cinnamon (optional, for flavor)

- Ice cubes (optional, for a colder smoothie)

Preparation:

1. Ensure the beetroot is cooked, cooled, and chopped into smaller pieces.

2. Add the cooked beetroot, mixed berries, Greek yogurt, almond milk, honey (if desired), and ground cinnamon (if using) to a blender.

3. If you prefer a colder smoothie, you can add a few ice cubes as well.

4. Blend all the ingredients until you achieve a smooth and creamy consistency.

5. If the smoothie is too thick, you can add more almond milk to reach your desired consistency.

6. Pour the Beetroot and Berry Smoothie into a glass.

7. Serve immediately and enjoy!

Nutritional Value (per serving):

- Calories: Approximately 200-250 (varies based on ingredients and sweetener)

- Carbohydrates: 40-50g

- Dietary Fiber: 7-9g

- Protein: 8-10g

- Vitamin C (from berries and beetroot): Provides a significant portion of the daily recommended intake

- Folate (from beetroot): Provides a significant portion of the daily recommended intake

Cooking Time: 5-10 minutes (depending on the preparation of the beetroot)

Rating: ★★★★★

A vibrant and nutritious smoothie that combines the earthy sweetness of beetroot with the fruity flavors of mixed berries. The addition of yogurt adds creaminess, making it a delicious and healthy choice for breakfast or a snack.

Cucumber and Mint Infused Water

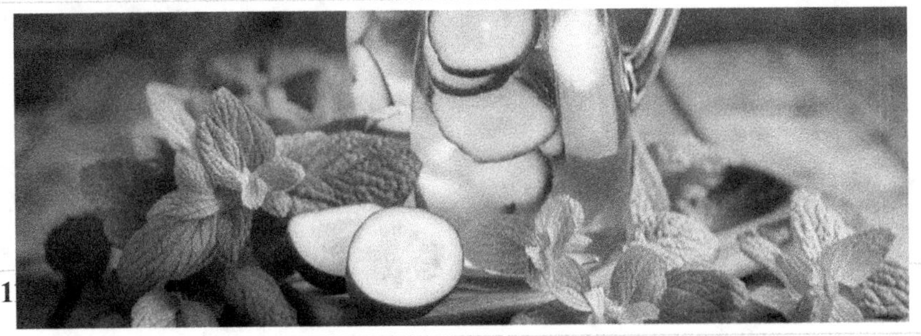

Ingredients:

- 1 cucumber, thinly sliced
- A handful of fresh mint leaves
- 8-10 cups of water
- Ice cubes (optional, for a colder drink)

Preparation:

1. Wash the cucumber thoroughly and slice it into thin rounds.

2. Rinse the fresh mint leaves.

3. In a large pitcher or jug, add the cucumber slices and fresh mint leaves.

4. Fill the pitcher with 8-10 cups of water.

5. If you prefer a colder infused water, you can add ice cubes to the pitcher.

6. Stir the ingredients gently to release their flavors.

7. Refrigerate the pitcher for at least 2 hours (or overnight) to allow the flavors to infuse.

8. Serve your refreshing Cucumber and Mint Infused Water in glasses, and you can refill the pitcher with more water as needed.

Nutritional Value (per serving):

- Calories: Approximately 0-5 (negligible)

- Carbohydrates: Negligible

- Dietary Fiber: Negligible

- Mint provides a small amount of vitamins and antioxidants.

Cooking Time: 5-10 minutes (mainly for slicing and assembling)

Rating: ★★★★★

A hydrating and flavorful beverage that's perfect for staying refreshed throughout the day. The combination of cool cucumber and fresh mint offers a delightful and soothing experience. It's a healthy alternative to sugary drinks.

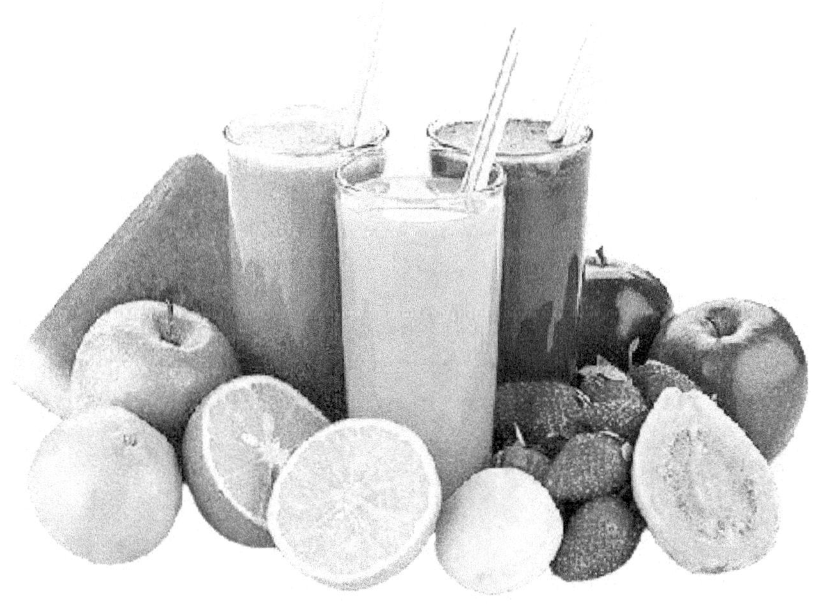

Appendix

Meal Plan Sample

Week 1:

Day 1:

- **Breakfast:** Oatmeal with Fresh Berries

- **Lunch:** Quinoa and Roasted Vegetable Salad

- **Dinner:** Baked Salmon with Steamed Broccoli

- **Snack:** Carrot and Cucumber Sticks with Hummus

Day 2:

- **Breakfast:** Spinach and Mushroom Egg White Omelette

- **Lunch:** Grilled Chicken with Mediterranean Salad

- **Dinner:** Grilled Turkey Breast with Quinoa Pilaf

- **Snack:** Fresh Fruit Salad

Day 3:

- **Breakfast:** Banana and Almond Milk Smoothie

- **Lunch:** Lentil Soup with Whole Grain Bread

- **Dinner:** Vegetable Lasagna with Ricotta Cheese

- **Snack:** Baked Kale Chips

Day 4:

- **Breakfast:** Whole Grain Avocado Toast

- **Lunch:** Tofu and Veggie Stir-Fry

- **Dinner:** Baked Sweet Potato with Sautéed Spinach

- **Snack:** Roasted Chickpeas

Day 5:

- **Breakfast:** Apple and Walnut Yogurt Parfait

- **Lunch:** Avocado and Turkey Wrap

- **Dinner:** Grilled Shrimp with Brown Rice and Asparagus

- **Snack:** Steamed Edamame with Sea Salt

Week 2:

Day 6:

- **Breakfast:** Oatmeal with Fresh Berries

- **Lunch:** Quinoa and Roasted Vegetable Salad

- **Dinner:** Baked Salmon with Steamed Broccoli

- **Snack:** Carrot and Cucumber Sticks with Hummus

Day 7:

- **Breakfast:** Spinach and Mushroom Egg White Omelette

- **Lunch:** Grilled Chicken with Mediterranean Salad

- **Dinner:** Grilled Turkey Breast with Quinoa Pilaf

- **Snack:** Fresh Fruit Salad

Day 8:

- **Breakfast:** Banana and Almond Milk Smoothie

- **Lunch:** Lentil Soup with Whole Grain Bread

- **Dinner:** Vegetable Lasagna with Ricotta Cheese

- **Snack:** Baked Kale Chips

Day 9:

- **Breakfast:** Whole Grain Avocado Toast

- **Lunch:** Tofu and Veggie Stir-Fry

- **Dinner:** Baked Sweet Potato with Sautéed Spinach

- **Snack:** Roasted Chickpeas

Day 10:

- **Breakfast:** Apple and Walnut Yogurt Parfait

- **Lunch:** Avocado and Turkey Wrap

- **Dinner:** Grilled Shrimp with Brown Rice and Asparagus

- **Snack:** Steamed Edamame with Sea Salt

Week 3:

Day 11:

- **Breakfast:** Oatmeal with Fresh Berries

- **Lunch:** Quinoa and Roasted Vegetable Salad

- **Dinner:** Baked Salmon with Steamed Broccoli

- **Snack:** Carrot and Cucumber Sticks with Hummus

Day 12:

- **Breakfast:** Spinach and Mushroom Egg White Omelette

- **Lunch:** Grilled Chicken with Mediterranean Salad

- **Dinner:** Grilled Turkey Breast with Quinoa Pilaf

- **Snack:** Fresh Fruit Salad

Day 13:

- **Breakfast:** Banana and Almond Milk Smoothie

- **Lunch:** Lentil Soup with Whole Grain Bread

- **Dinner:** Vegetable Lasagna with Ricotta Cheese

- **Snack:** Baked Kale Chips

Day 14:

- **Breakfast:** Whole Grain Avocado Toast

- **Lunch:** Tofu and Veggie Stir-Fry

- **Dinner:** Baked Sweet Potato with Sautéed Spinach

- **Snack:** Roasted Chickpeas

Day 15:

- **Breakfast:** Apple and Walnut Yogurt Parfait

- **Lunch:** Avocado and Turkey Wrap

- **Dinner:** Grilled Shrimp with Brown Rice and Asparagus

- **Snack:** Steamed Edamame with Sea Salt

Week 4:

Day 16:

- **Breakfast:** Oatmeal with Fresh Berries

- **Lunch:** Quinoa and Roasted Vegetable Salad

- **Dinner:** Baked Salmon with Steamed Broccoli

- **Snack:** Carrot and Cucumber Sticks with Hummus

Day 17:

- **Breakfast:** Spinach and Mushroom Egg White Omelette

- **Lunch:** Grilled Chicken with Mediterranean Salad

- **Dinner:** Grilled Turkey Breast with Quinoa Pilaf

- **Snack:** Fresh Fruit Salad

Day 18:

- **Breakfast:** Banana and Almond Milk Smoothie

- **Lunch:** Lentil Soup with Whole Grain Bread

- **Dinner:** Vegetable Lasagna with Ricotta Cheese

- **Snack:** Baked Kale Chips

Day 19:

- **Breakfast:** Whole Grain Avocado Toast

- **Lunch:** Tofu and Veggie Stir-Fry

- **Dinner:** Baked Sweet Potato with Sautéed Spinach

- **Snack:** Roasted Chickpeas

Day 20:

- **Breakfast:** Apple and Walnut Yogurt Parfait

- **Lunch:** Avocado and Turkey Wrap

- **Dinner:** Grilled Shrimp with Brown Rice and Asparagus

- **Snack:** Steamed Edamame with Sea Salt

Throughout the month, you can enjoy various soups, meat and poultry dishes, seafood and fish, and delicious desserts. Don't forget to stay hydrated with your choice of beverages, such as Green Tea with Lemon, Ginger and Turmeric Herbal Tea, Fresh Carrot and Apple Juice, and Beetroot and Berry Smoothie.

Remember to adjust portion sizes and ingredients to fit your dietary preferences and needs. Enjoy your month of wholesome and delicious meals!

Meal Planning and Prepping for Liver Health

Planning and preparing meals for liver health is essential for anybody hoping to sustain and improve liver function. Getting the appropriate nutrients and avoiding bad meals is crucial for the liver since it is responsible for both detoxifying the body and digesting nutrition. This is how to prepare and plan meals for the health of your liver:

1. Include Foods Good for Liver Function:

Leafy Greens: Include veggies that aid in detoxifying and are high in antioxidants, such as broccoli, kale, and spinach.

Cruciferous vegetables: These are good for liver enzymes and include cabbage, cauliflower, and Brussels sprouts.

Healthy Fats: Choose foods high in essential fatty acids that support liver function, such as avocados, almonds, and seeds.

Lean Proteins: To lessen the strain on your liver, choose lean protein sources like chicken, turkey, fish, and tofu.

High-Fiber Foods: Rich in fiber, fruits, legumes, and whole grains help to maintain digestive health and stave against fatty liver disease.

2. Minimize Dangerous Substances:

Minimize Alcohol: Drinking too much alcohol can harm your liver, so cut back on it or avoid it altogether.

Eat Less Processed Meals: Trans fats, preservatives, and additives found in processed meals can be harmful to the liver.

Limit Sugar Intake: Consuming sugary drinks and snacks should be avoided as it might lead to fatty liver disease.

Control Sodium: Too much salt can cause liver problems and fluid retention, so watch what you eat.

3. Well-Composed Meals:

Make sure you eat a selection of food categories in your well-balanced meals to ensure you are getting a variety of nutrients.

4. Meal Planning Advice:

Cook in groups: Make many portions of foods that are good for the liver and freeze them.

Portion control: To prevent overindulging, use portion-sized containers.

Date and label: To maintain freshness, make sure your meal preparation goods are properly labeled and dated.

Include liver-supporting elements in your dishes, such as ginger, garlic, and turmeric.

5. Choose Your Snacks Carefully:

To satisfy your desires, choose nutritious snacks like unsalted almonds, fresh fruit, or carrot sticks with hummus.

6. Maintain Hydration:

Drink plenty of water throughout the day to help your body rid itself of pollutants.

7. Examine Add-ons:

Before using any supplements or herbal therapies to promote liver health, speak with your healthcare physician.

8. Track Your Development:

Make sure your liver health is improving by scheduling frequent check-ups with a medical practitioner and having the required tests carried out.

9. Look for Expert Advice:

For individualized guidance, speak with a trained dietitian or your healthcare physician if you have any concerns or problems related to your liver.

Recall that eating well is only one aspect of a diet that supports liver function; there are other important factors as well. To promote the health of your liver and entire body, give priority to fresh, complete foods and incorporate meal planning and preparation into your daily routine.

Healthy Cooking Techniques

Healthy cooking skills are vital for treating fatty liver and cirrhosis since they assist in minimizing liver strain, inflammation, and general liver health. Here are several cooking methods to consider:

1. Grilling or Broiling:

Grilling and broiling are excellent ways to prepare lean foods such as chicken, turkey, fish, and tofu without adding unnecessary fat. Marinate in herbs and spices for taste.

2. Baking and Roasting:

Baking and roasting vegetables, lean meats, and fish may improve their flavor and texture without using excessive oil or fat.

3. Steaming:

Steaming veggies, such as broccoli and cauliflower, preserve their nutrients while making them more digestible.

4. Sauté and Stir-fry:

Sauté and stir-fry using tiny amounts of heart-healthy oils such as olive or avocado oil. Maintain a moderate heat to avoid excessive browning.

5. Poaching.

Poaching delicate meats such as fish and poultry in flavorful broth or water is a gentle cooking method that keeps them moist.

6. Boiling:

Whole grains such as brown rice, quinoa, and whole wheat pasta can be prepared by boiling them. It helps preserve their original tastes.

7. Seasoning with Herbs and Spices

Instead of salt, season your foods with herbs and spices such as turmeric, ginger, garlic, and rosemary. These may have anti-inflammatory qualities and provide dimension to your meals.

Healthy cooking skills not only benefit liver health but also improve general well-being. They can help control fatty liver and cirrhosis by lowering inflammation and delivering nutrients that your liver requires to operate properly.

Managing Dietary Restrictions and Allergies

Managing dietary restrictions and allergies when treating cirrhosis and fatty liver is critical to ensuring sufficient nutrition while protecting your liver. Here are some guidelines for dealing with these conditions:

1. Consult with A Healthcare Provider:

Collaborate with your healthcare practitioner and a trained dietitian to create a tailored meal plan that addresses your unique dietary restrictions and allergies.

2. Identify Food Allergies and Intolerances:

Determine whether you have any food allergies or intolerances and avoid them totally. Common allergies include dairy, gluten, soy, and nuts.

3. Focus on Whole Foods:

Include complete, unprocessed foods in your diet. This includes fruits and vegetables, lean proteins, entire grains, and legumes. These foods are typically suitable for most dietary restrictions.

4. Avoid Trigger Foods.

Identify and avoid foods that worsen your symptoms or allergies. For example, if you are lactose intolerant, select lactose-free dairy alternatives.

5. Customize Recipes:

Modify recipes to suit your nutritional requirements. If you have celiac disease, substitute wheat-based items with gluten-free equivalents.

6. Read Labels Carefully.

Read food labels to detect potential allergies and substances that may be incompatible with your condition. Look for "free-from" alternatives when they're available.

7. Substitute Ingredients:

Replace problematic components with acceptable substitutes. If you are lactose-sensitive, you can use almond milk instead of cow's milk.

9. Limit Sodium Intake:

Limit your salt intake, particularly if you have cirrhosis, to avoid fluid retention. Avoid processed and salty meals.

9. Manage Portion Sizes.

Avoid overeating, which can strain your liver, by keeping portion sizes in check. Use smaller plates and utensils to improve portion control.

10. Stay hydrated: - Consume plenty of fluids, particularly water, to keep hydrated and help your liver work properly.

11. Monitor Protein Consumption: - If you have cirrhosis, limit your protein consumption as excess might be harmful. A licensed dietitian can assist you in determining the appropriate protein intake for your specific needs.

12. Individualized Approach: - Understand that dietary limitations and allergies are unique to each individual. What works for one person may not work for others.

13. Supplements and Drugs: - Consult your healthcare professional if you require any supplements or drugs to treat particular deficiencies or symptoms.

14. Schedule frequent check-ups with your healthcare practitioner to monitor your condition and change your diet as necessary.

15. Seek Support: - Join support groups or connect with people with similar dietary limitations or liver issues. They can provide significant insights and guidance.

Remember that maintaining dietary restrictions and allergies while treating cirrhosis and fatty liver needs meticulous planning and monitoring. Prioritizing your health is critical, and engaging with healthcare experts may give you the advice and assistance you need to implement a successful dietary management strategy.

Essential Glossary Shopping List

Creating a shopping list for treating cirrhosis and fatty liver should focus on liver-friendly and nutrient-rich foods while avoiding items that can exacerbate these conditions. Here's an essential glossary shopping list to help you plan your meals:

Proteins:

- Lean poultry (chicken, turkey)
- Fish (salmon, trout, tilapia)
- Tofu
- Legumes (lentils, chickpeas)
- Eggs (if well-tolerated)

Grains:

- Whole grains (brown rice, quinoa, whole wheat pasta)
- Oats
- Barley

Fruits:

- Berries (blueberries, strawberries, raspberries)

- Apples

- Citrus fruits (oranges, lemons, limes)

- Bananas

- Avocado

Vegetables:

- Leafy greens (spinach, kale, arugula)

- Cruciferous vegetables (broccoli, cauliflower, Brussels sprouts)

- Bell peppers

- Carrots

- Beets

- Cucumbers

- Zucchini

- Tomatoes

- Onions

- Garlic

Dairy and Dairy Alternatives (if tolerated):

- Greek yogurt (low-fat)

- Lactose-free milk

- Almond milk (unsweetened)

- Coconut milk (unsweetened)

Healthy Fats:

- Avocado

- Nuts (almonds, walnuts)

- Seeds (chia seeds, flaxseeds)

- Olive oil (extra-virgin)

Herbs and Spices:

- Turmeric

- Thyme

- Ginger

- Cilantro

- Garlic

- Parsley

- Rosemary

Beverages:

- Green tea

- Fresh carrot and apple juice (homemade)

- Herbal teas (ginger, peppermint, chamomile)

- Water (stay well-hydrated)

Condiments and Flavorings:

- Lemon juice

- Low-sodium soy sauce or tamari

- Balsamic vinegar

- Honey (in moderation)

- Mustard (Dijon or whole-grain)

- Spices (cinnamon, cumin, paprika)

Snacks and Treats (in moderation):

- Fresh fruit
- Nuts (portion-controlled)
- Baked kale chips
- Dark chocolate (high cocoa content)

Canned and Packaged Goods (low sodium):

- Low-sodium broths
- Canned vegetables (without added salt)
- Canned beans (rinsed and drained)
- Whole grain crackers (low-sodium)

Avoid or Limit:

- Alcohol
- Processed foods (chips, sugary snacks)
- Excessive salt (high-sodium processed foods)
- Red meat
- Sugary beverages
- Foods high in trans fats (fried foods)

Remember to check food labels for sodium content and avoid items high in added sugars and unhealthy fats. Tailor your shopping list to your specific dietary needs and preferences, and consult with a healthcare provider or dietitian for personalized guidance on managing cirrhosis and fatty liver through nutrition.

For further Questions and advice reach out on

joanmilonehelpdesk@gmail.com

Thank You

I'm writing this with a heart full of gratitude for your kind words and the time you took to read my book, knowing that my words have resonated with you is a reward beyond measure. Thank you again for your appreciation and for being a part of this literary journey.

Warmly,

Joan

>>> 30 Days Meal Planner

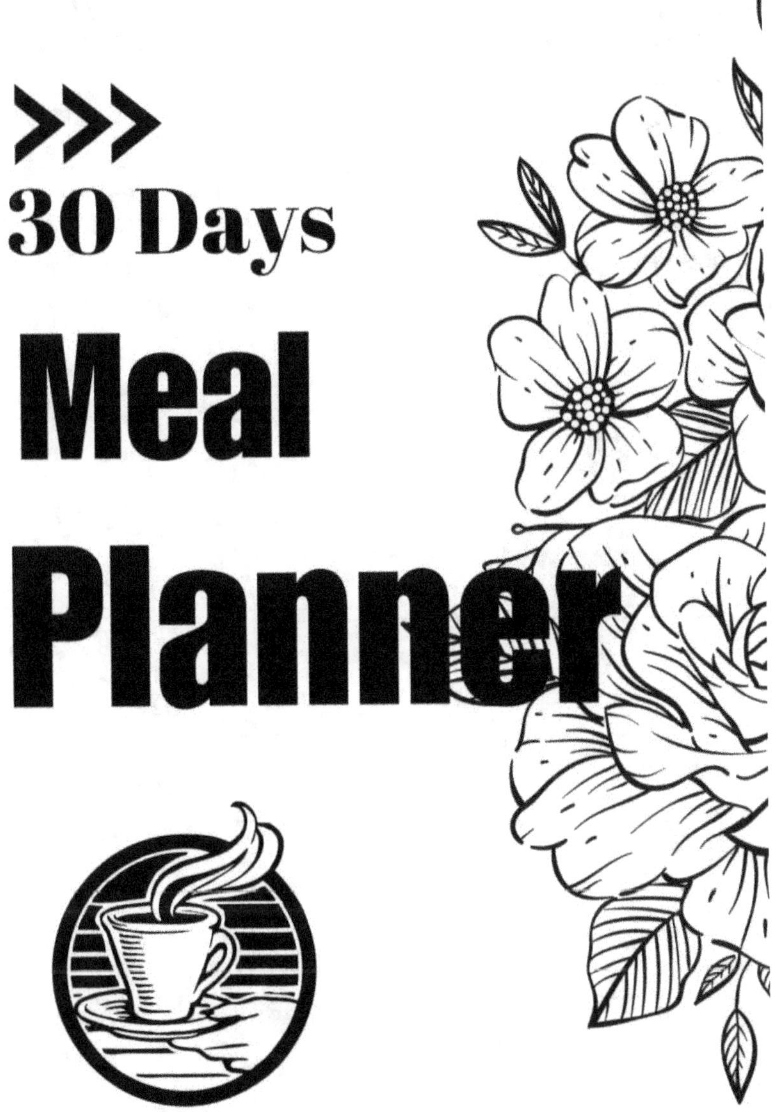

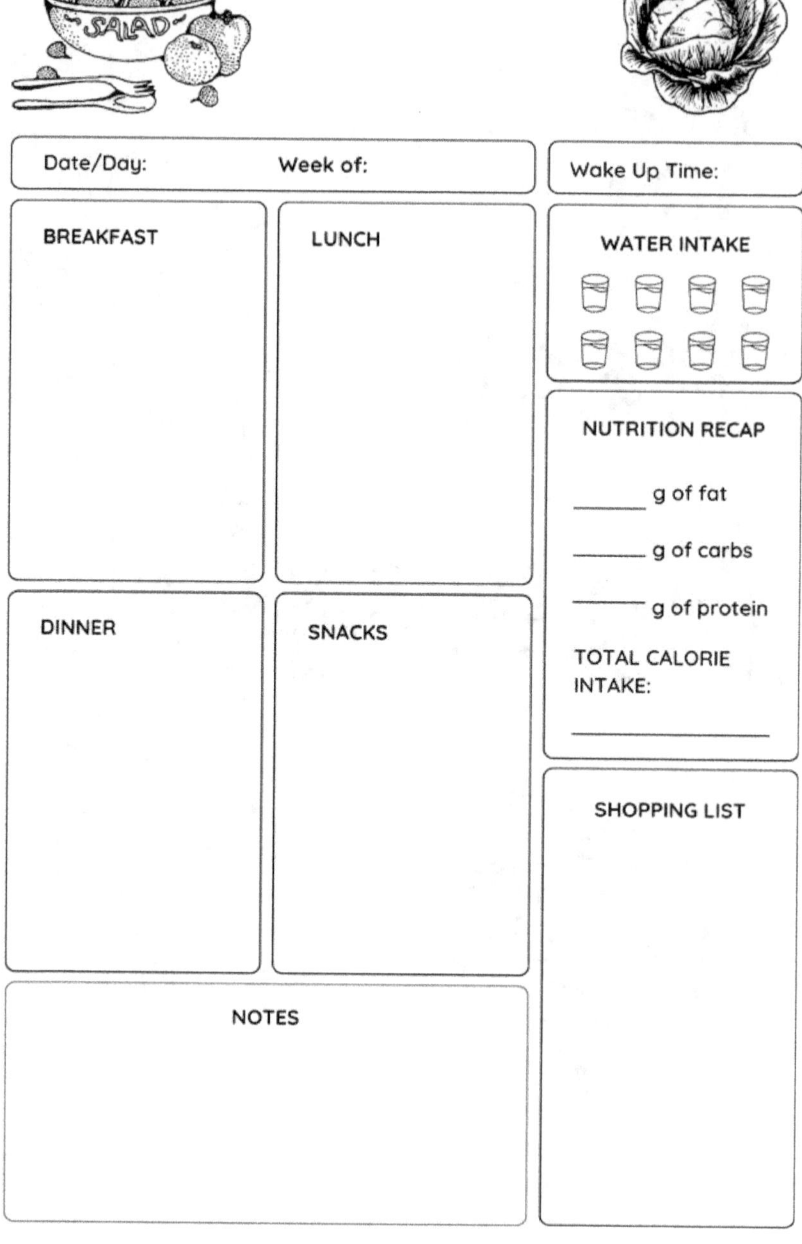

Date/Day:
Week of:
Wake Up Time:
BREAKFAST
LUNCH
WATER INTAKE
NUTRITION RECAP
_______ g of fat
_______ g of carbs
_______ g of protein
TOTAL CALORIE INTAKE:
DINNER
SNACKS
SHOPPING LIST
NOTES

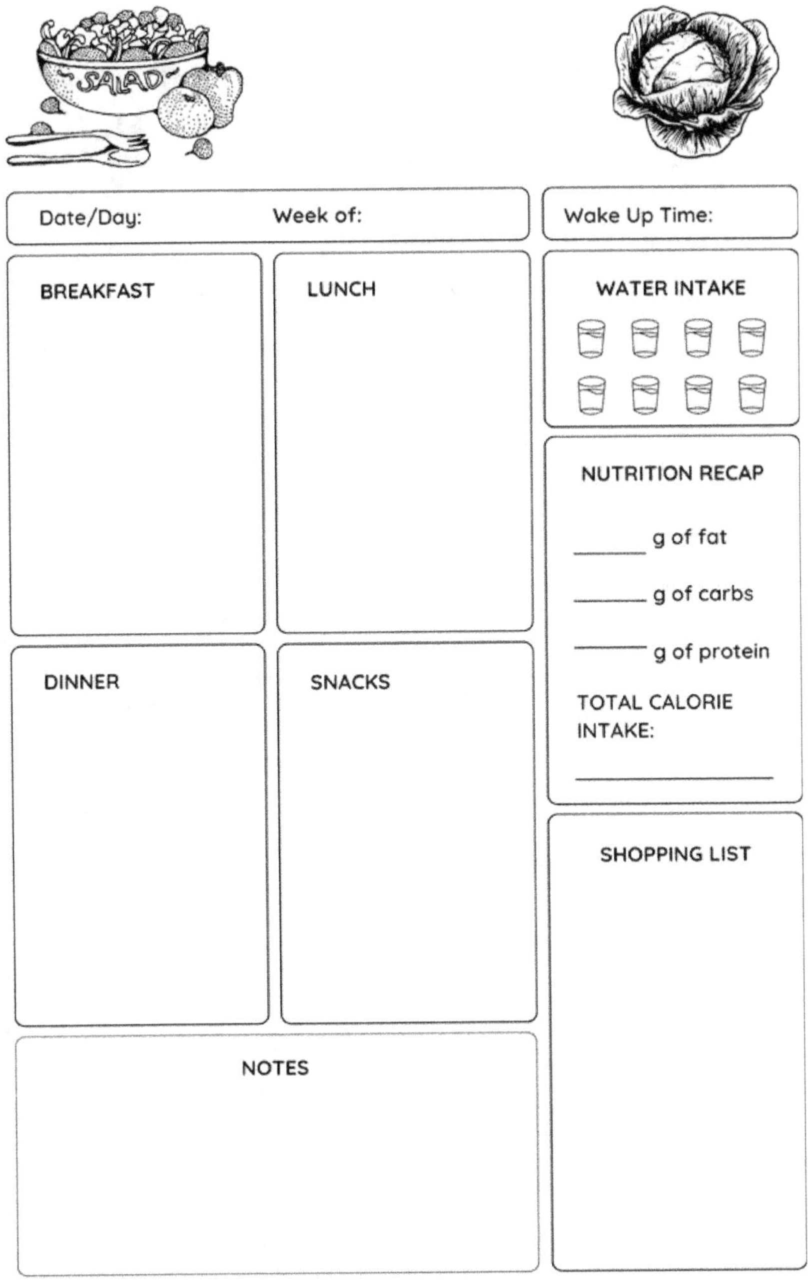

Date/Day:
Week of:
Wake Up Time:
BREAKFAST
LUNCH
WATER INTAKE
NUTRITION RECAP
_______ g of fat
_______ g of carbs
_______ g of protein
TOTAL CALORIE INTAKE:
DINNER
SNACKS
SHOPPING LIST
NOTES

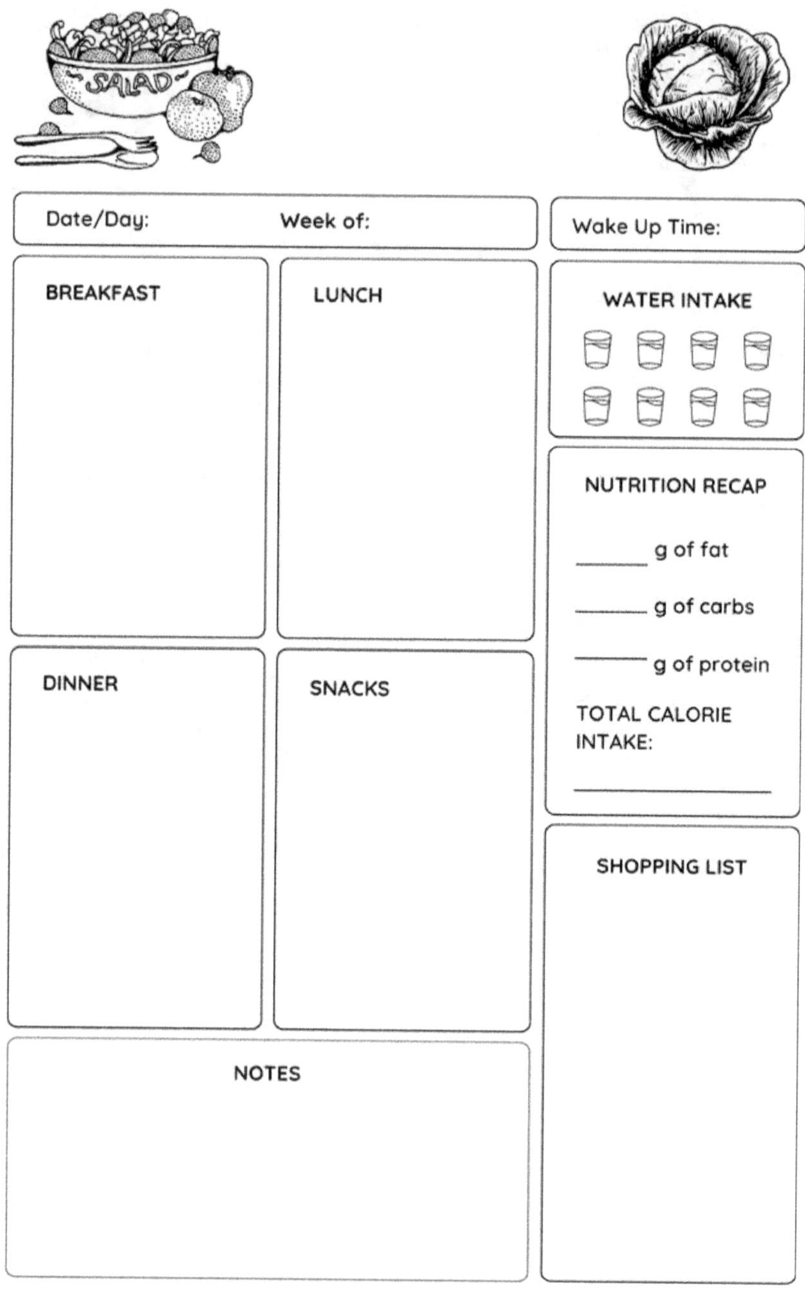

Date/Day: Week of:

Wake Up Time:

BREAKFAST

LUNCH

WATER INTAKE

NUTRITION RECAP

_________ g of fat

_________ g of carbs

_________ g of protein

TOTAL CALORIE INTAKE:

____

DINNER

SNACKS

SHOPPING LIST

NOTES

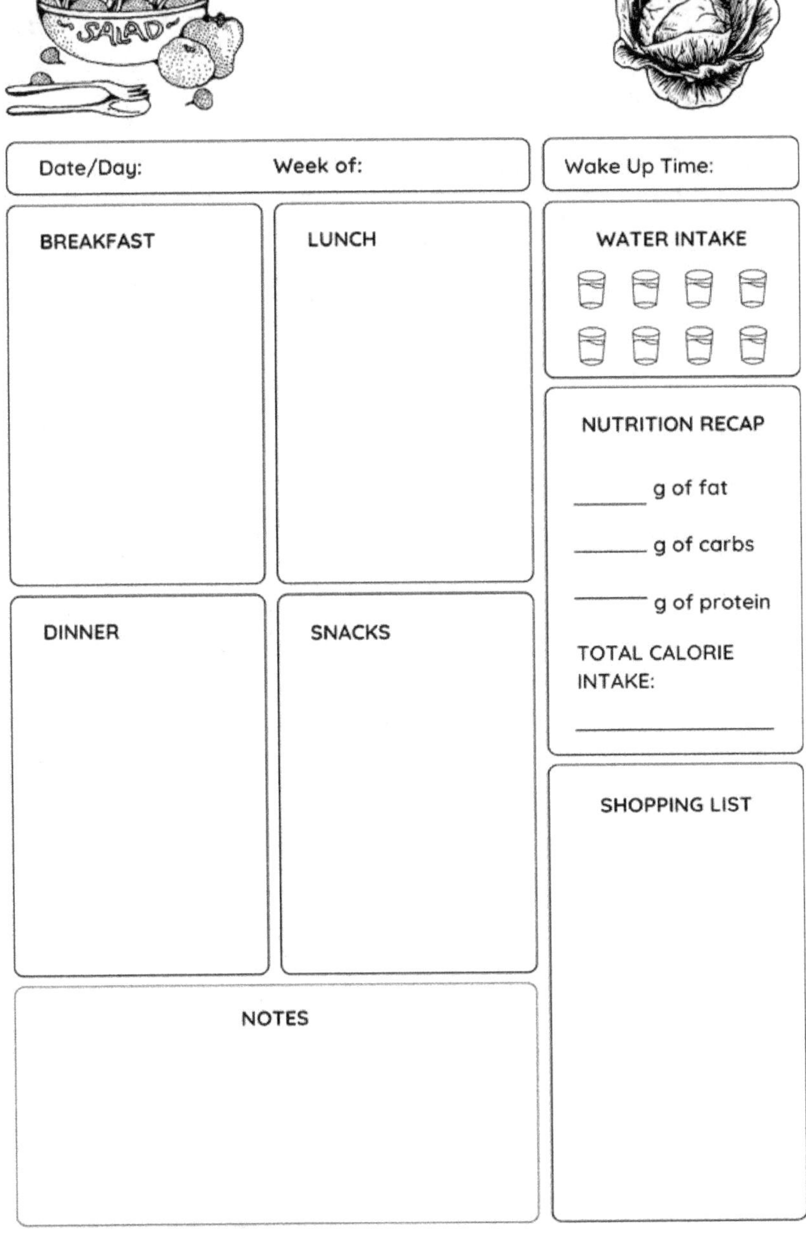

| Date/Day: | Week of: | Wake Up Time: |

BREAKFAST

LUNCH

WATER INTAKE

NUTRITION RECAP

_______ g of fat

_______ g of carbs

_______ g of protein

TOTAL CALORIE INTAKE:

____

DINNER

SNACKS

SHOPPING LIST

NOTES

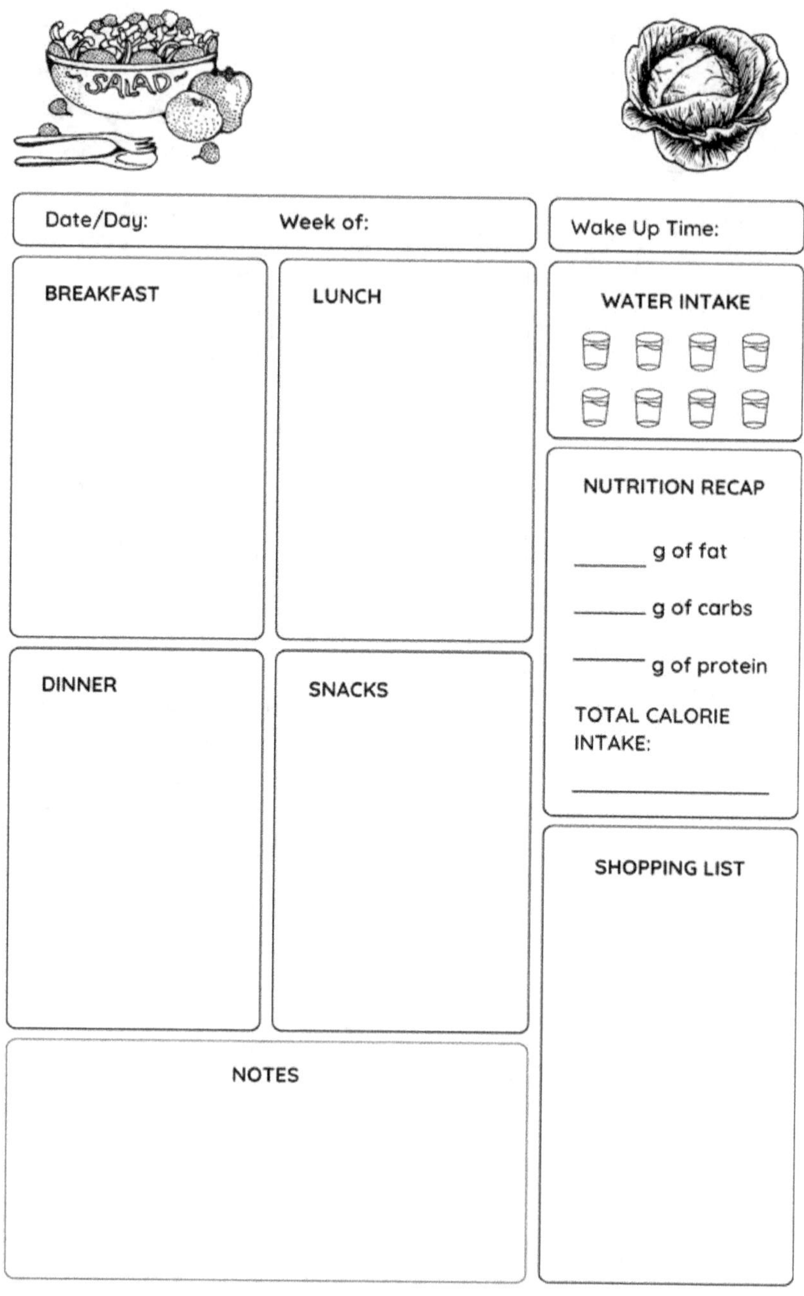

| Date/Day: | Week of: | Wake Up Time: |

BREAKFAST

LUNCH

WATER INTAKE

NUTRITION RECAP

_______ g of fat

_______ g of carbs

_______ g of protein

TOTAL CALORIE INTAKE:

____

DINNER

SNACKS

SHOPPING LIST

NOTES

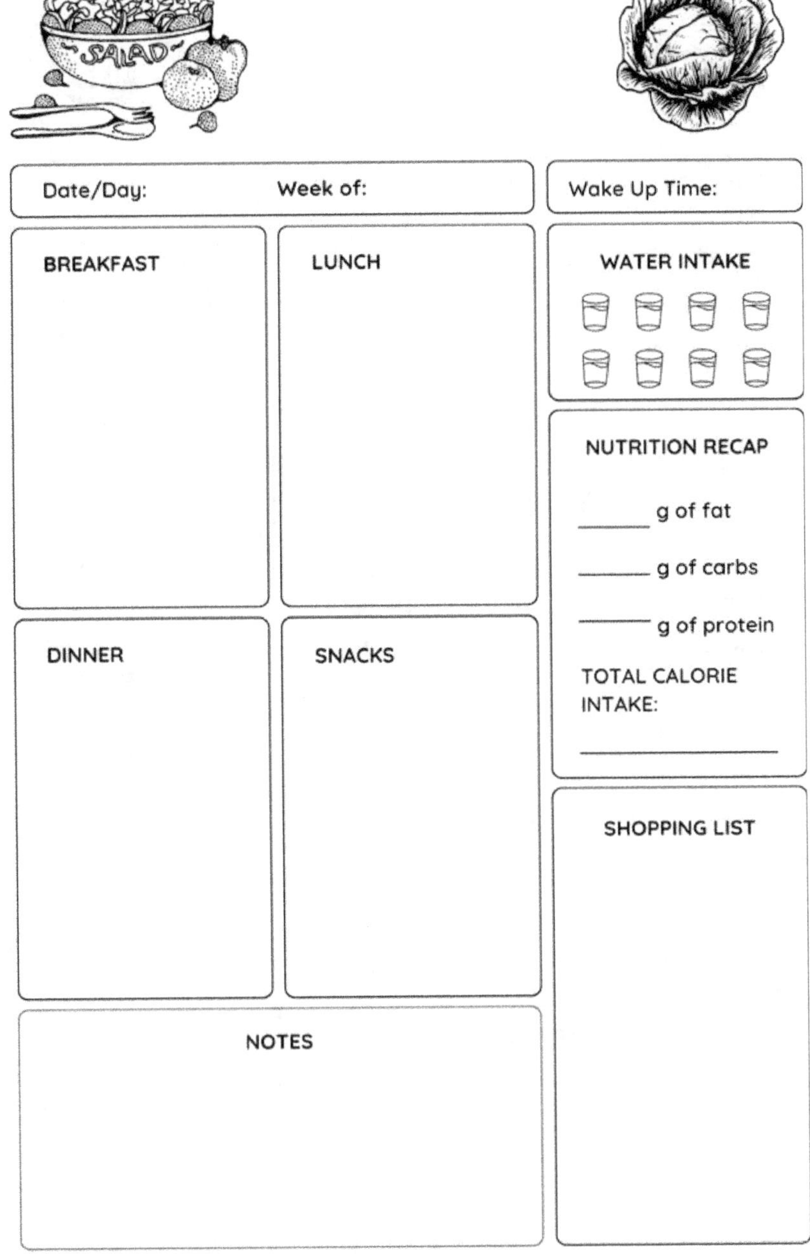

Date/Day:
Week of:
Wake Up Time:
BREAKFAST
LUNCH
WATER INTAKE
NUTRITION RECAP
_______ g of fat
_______ g of carbs
_______ g of protein
TOTAL CALORIE INTAKE:
____
DINNER
SNACKS
SHOPPING LIST
NOTES

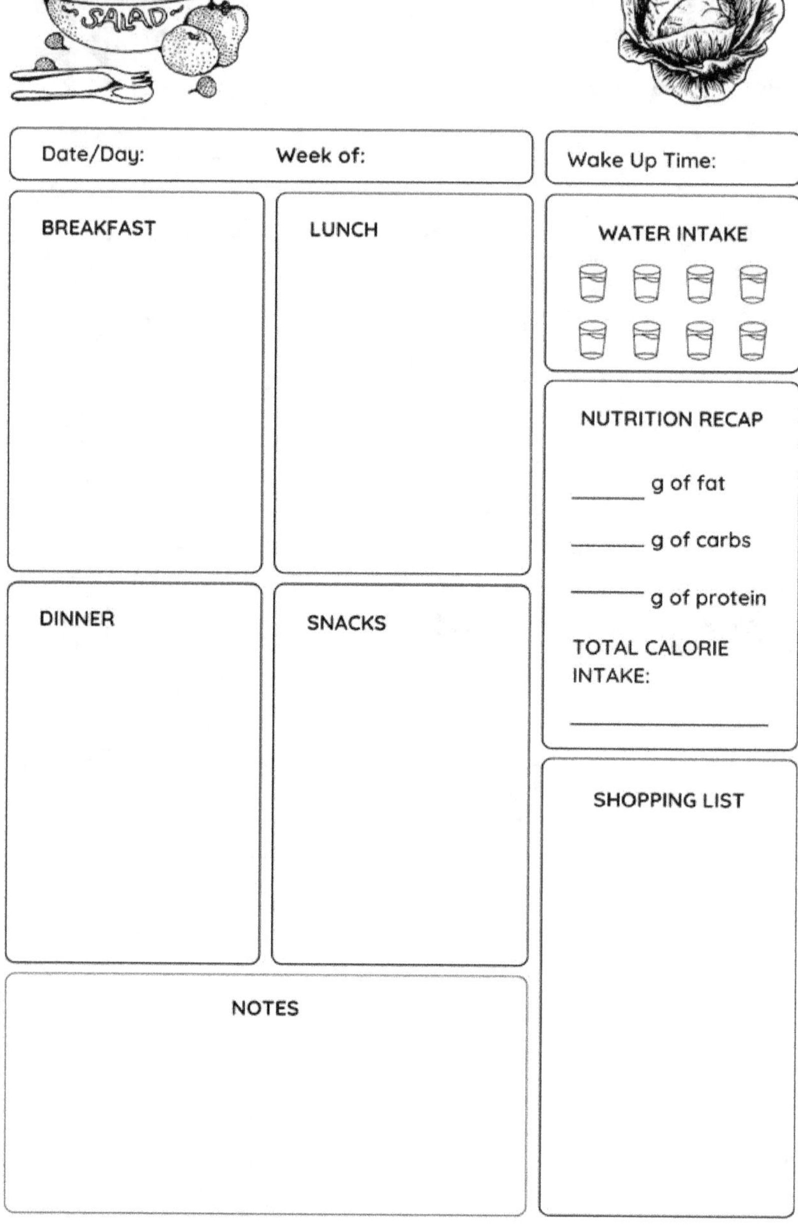

Date/Day:
Week of:
Wake Up Time:
BREAKFAST
LUNCH
WATER INTAKE
NUTRITION RECAP
_______ g of fat
_______ g of carbs
_______ g of protein
TOTAL CALORIE
INTAKE:
____
DINNER
SNACKS
SHOPPING LIST
NOTES

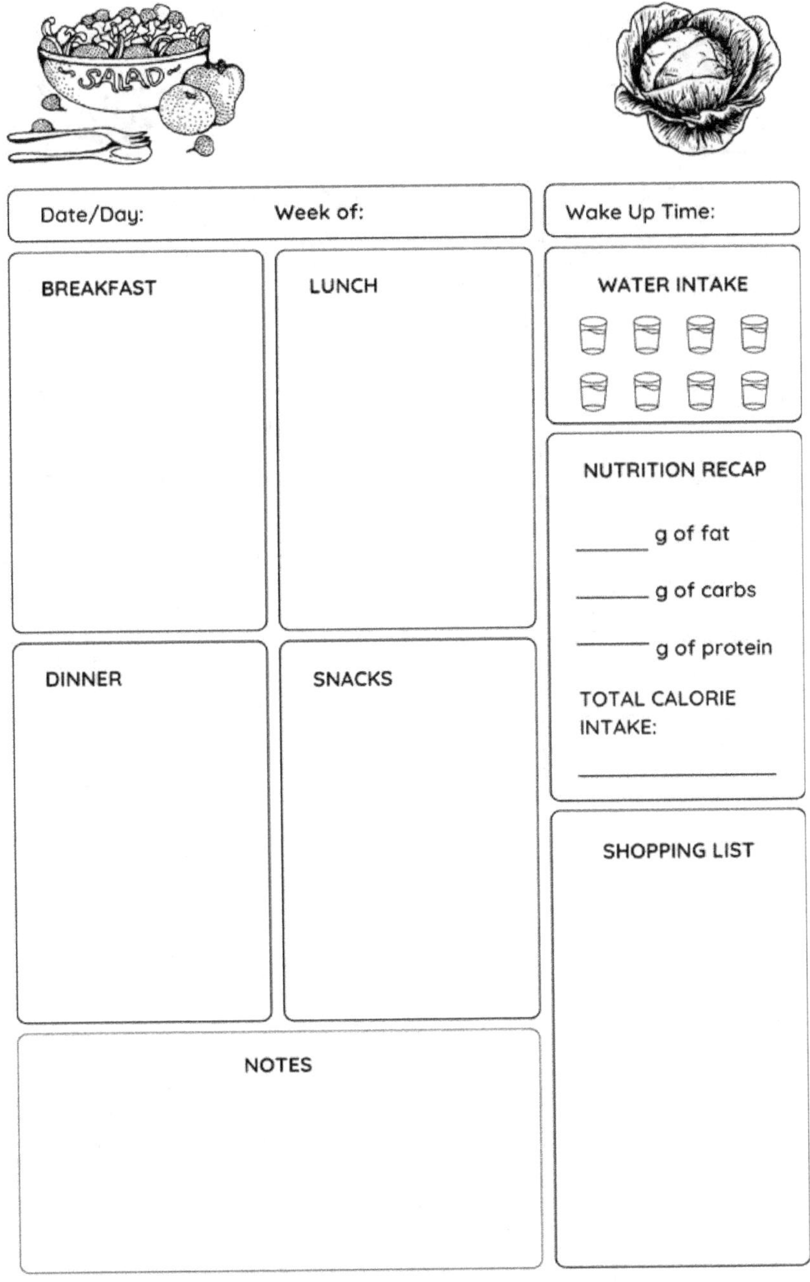
Date/Day:
Week of:
Wake Up Time:
BREAKFAST
LUNCH
WATER INTAKE
NUTRITION RECAP
_______ g of fat
_______ g of carbs
_______ g of protein
TOTAL CALORIE INTAKE:
DINNER
SNACKS
SHOPPING LIST
NOTES

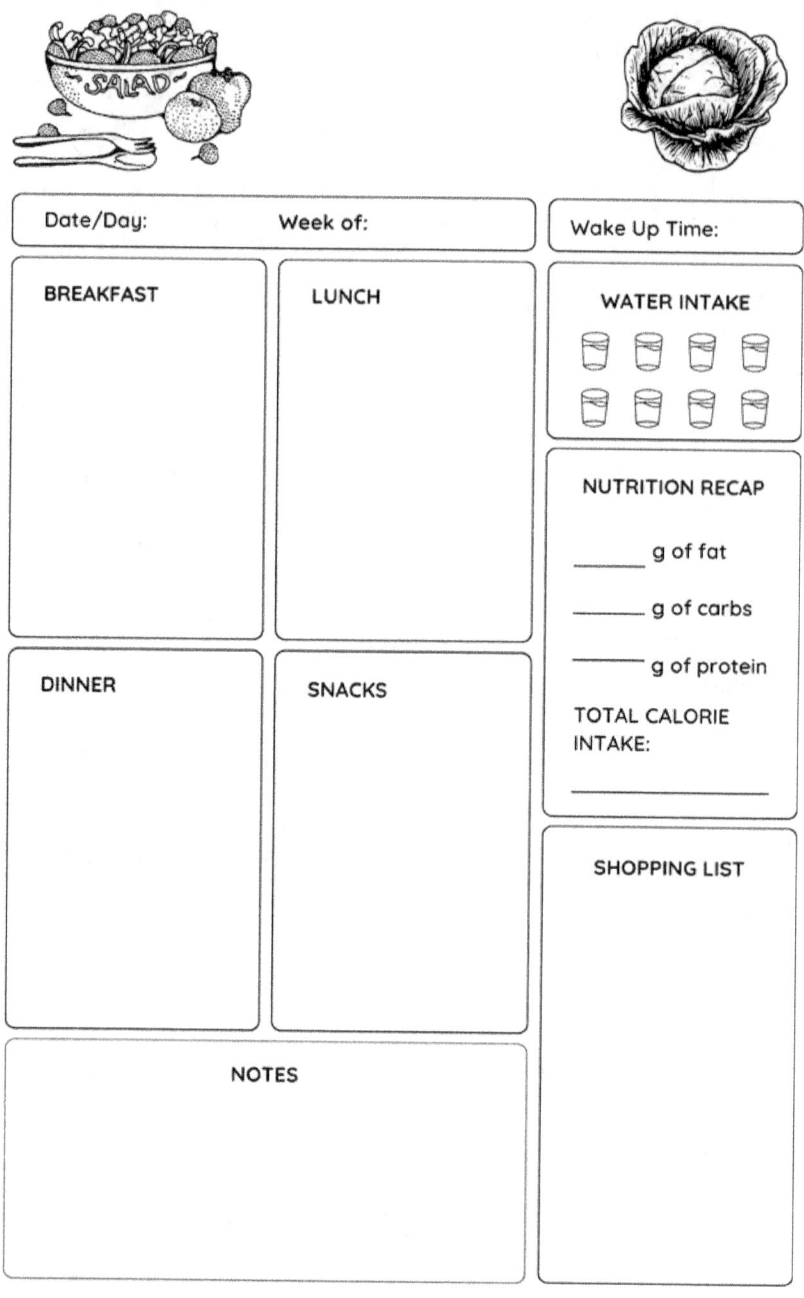

| Date/Day: | Week of: | Wake Up Time: |

BREAKFAST

LUNCH

WATER INTAKE

NUTRITION RECAP

_________ g of fat

_________ g of carbs

_________ g of protein

TOTAL CALORIE INTAKE:

____

DINNER

SNACKS

SHOPPING LIST

NOTES

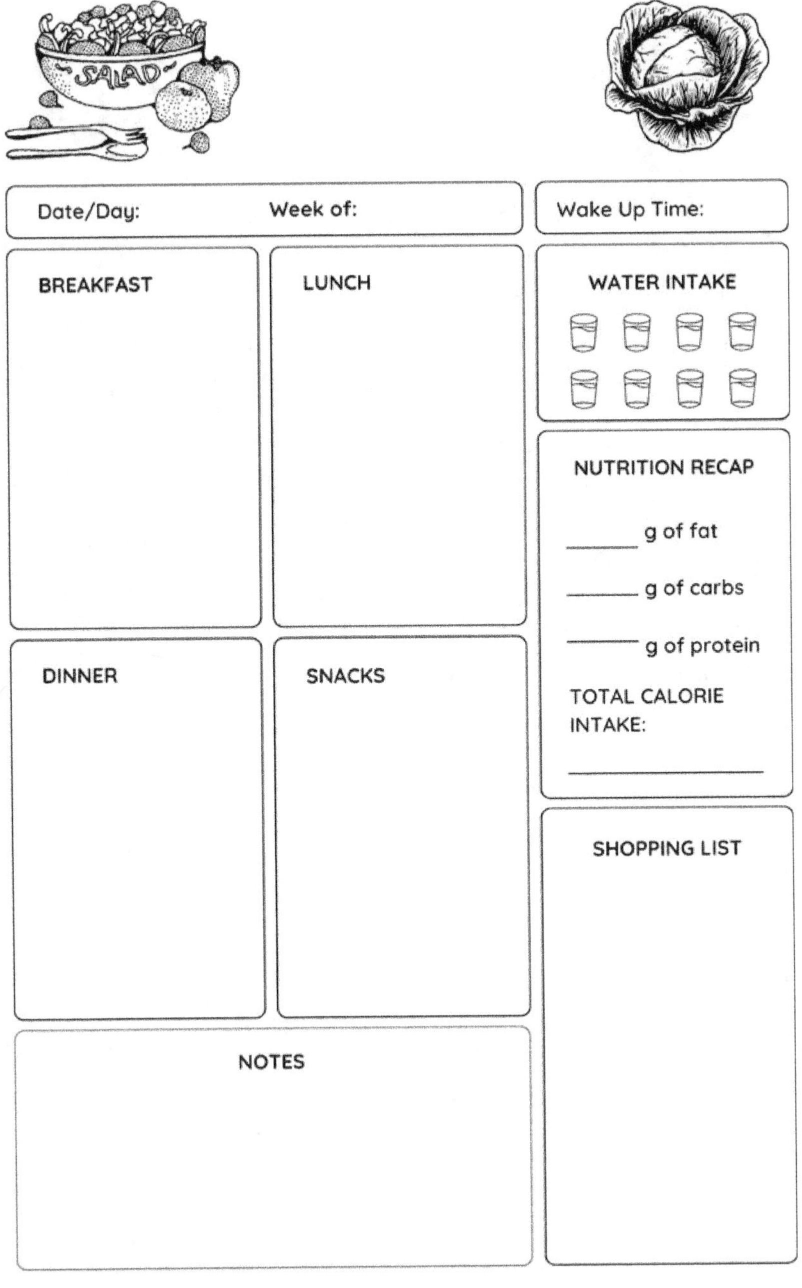

Date/Day:
Week of:
Wake Up Time:
BREAKFAST
LUNCH
WATER INTAKE
NUTRITION RECAP
_______ g of fat
_______ g of carbs
_______ g of protein
TOTAL CALORIE INTAKE:
DINNER
SNACKS
SHOPPING LIST
NOTES

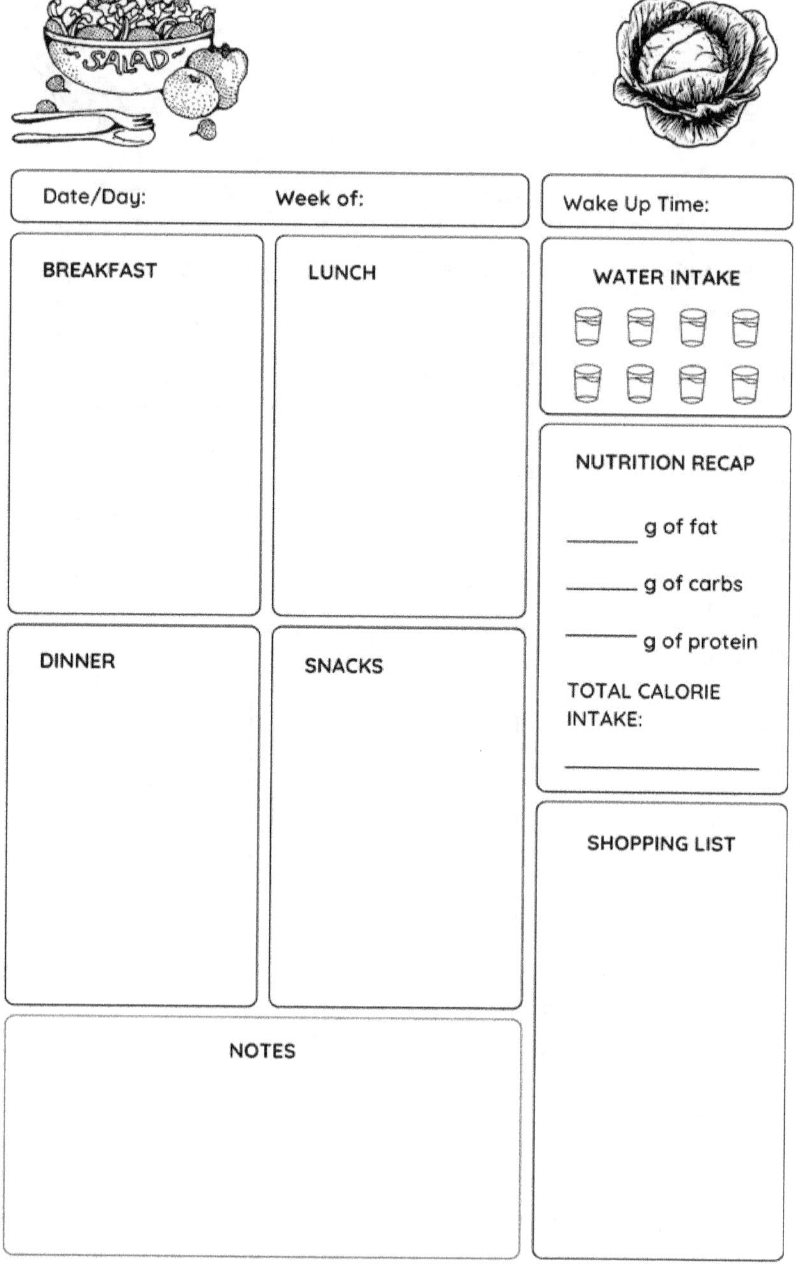

Date/Day:
Week of:
Wake Up Time:
BREAKFAST
LUNCH
WATER INTAKE
NUTRITION RECAP
_______ g of fat
_______ g of carbs
_______ g of protein
TOTAL CALORIE INTAKE:
DINNER
SNACKS
SHOPPING LIST
NOTES

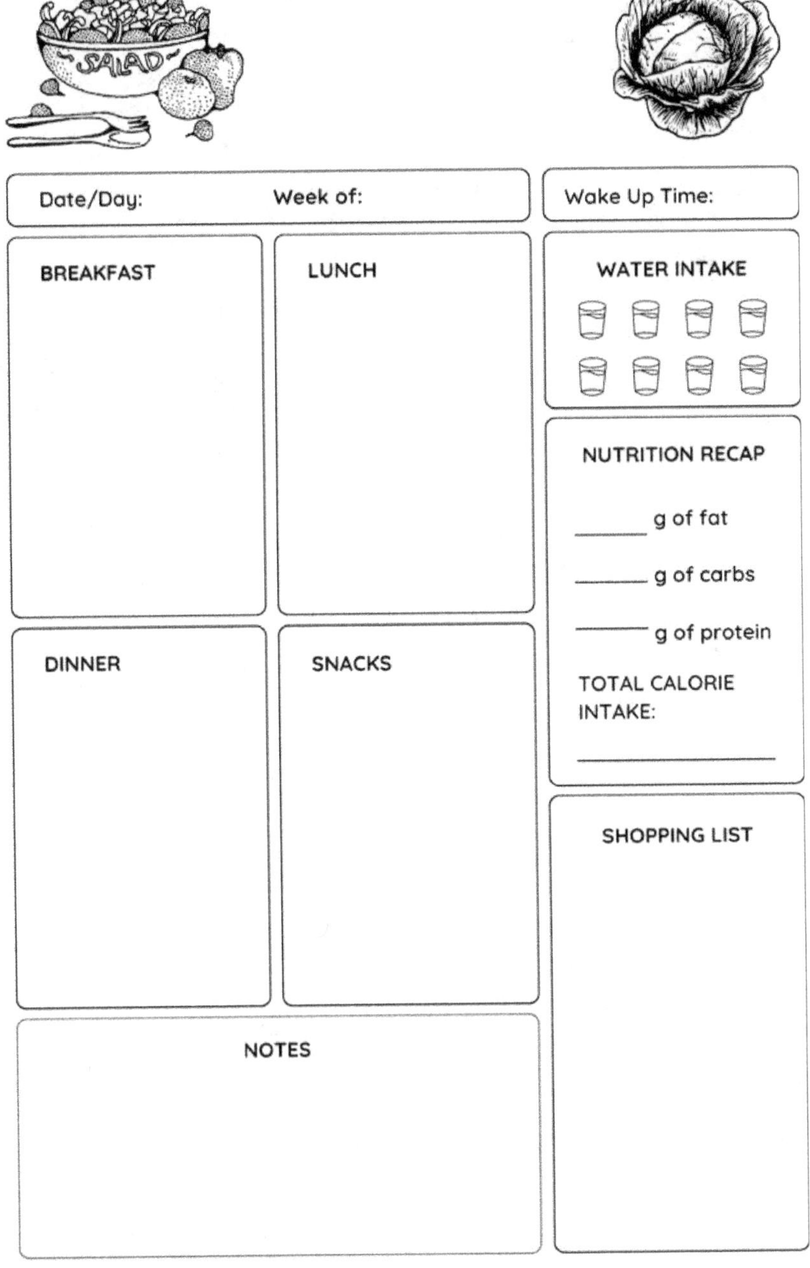
Date/Day:
Week of:
Wake Up Time:
BREAKFAST
LUNCH
WATER INTAKE
NUTRITION RECAP
_______ g of fat
_______ g of carbs
_______ g of protein
TOTAL CALORIE INTAKE:
DINNER
SNACKS
SHOPPING LIST
NOTES

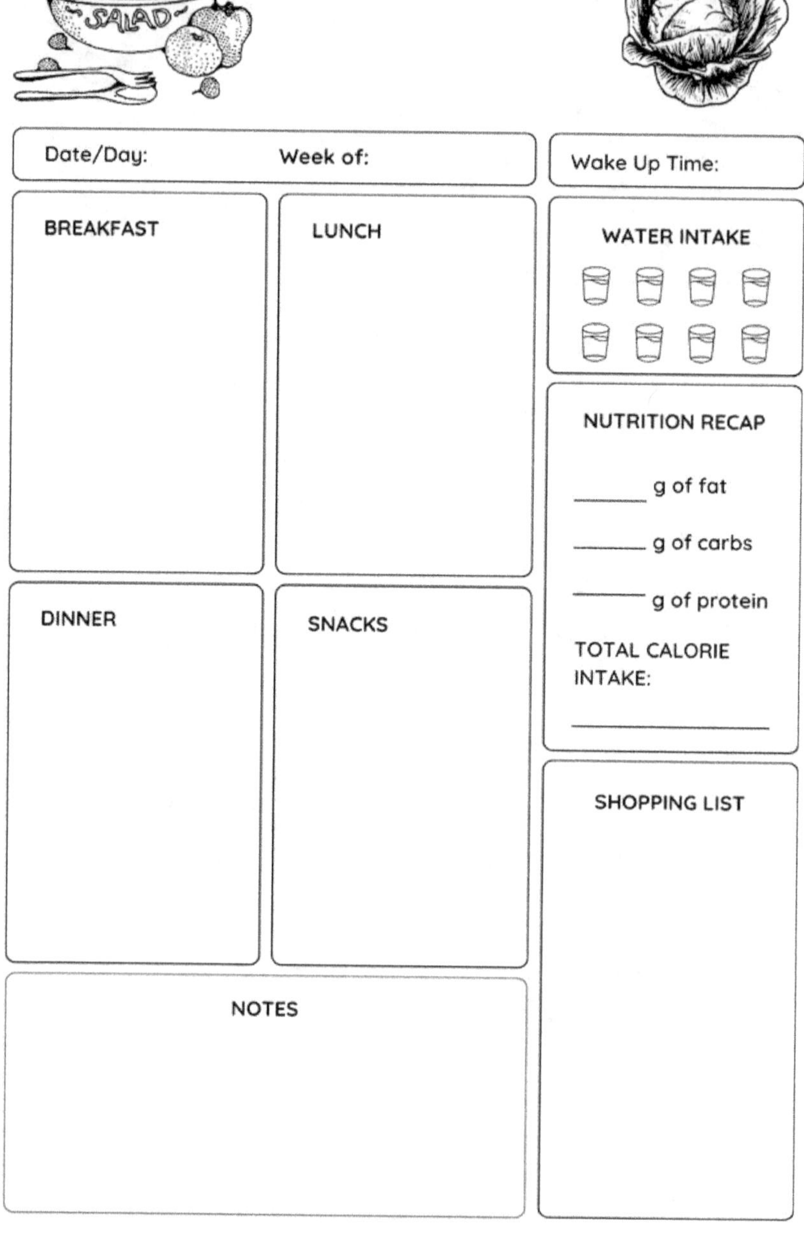

| Date/Day: | Week of: | Wake Up Time: |

BREAKFAST

LUNCH

WATER INTAKE

NUTRITION RECAP

______ g of fat

______ g of carbs

______ g of protein

TOTAL CALORIE INTAKE:

DINNER

SNACKS

SHOPPING LIST

NOTES

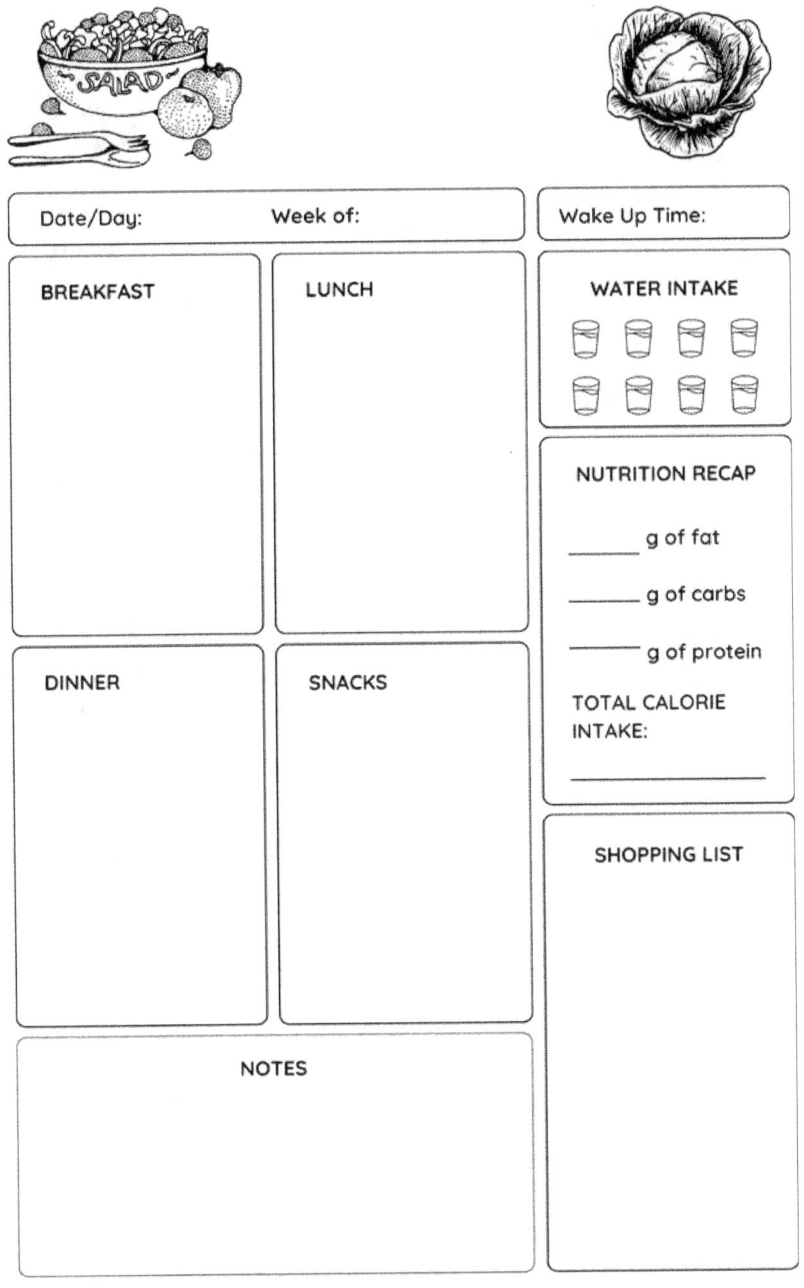

| Date/Day: | Week of: | Wake Up Time: |

BREAKFAST

LUNCH

WATER INTAKE

NUTRITION RECAP

_______ g of fat

_______ g of carbs

_______ g of protein

TOTAL CALORIE INTAKE:

____

DINNER

SNACKS

SHOPPING LIST

NOTES

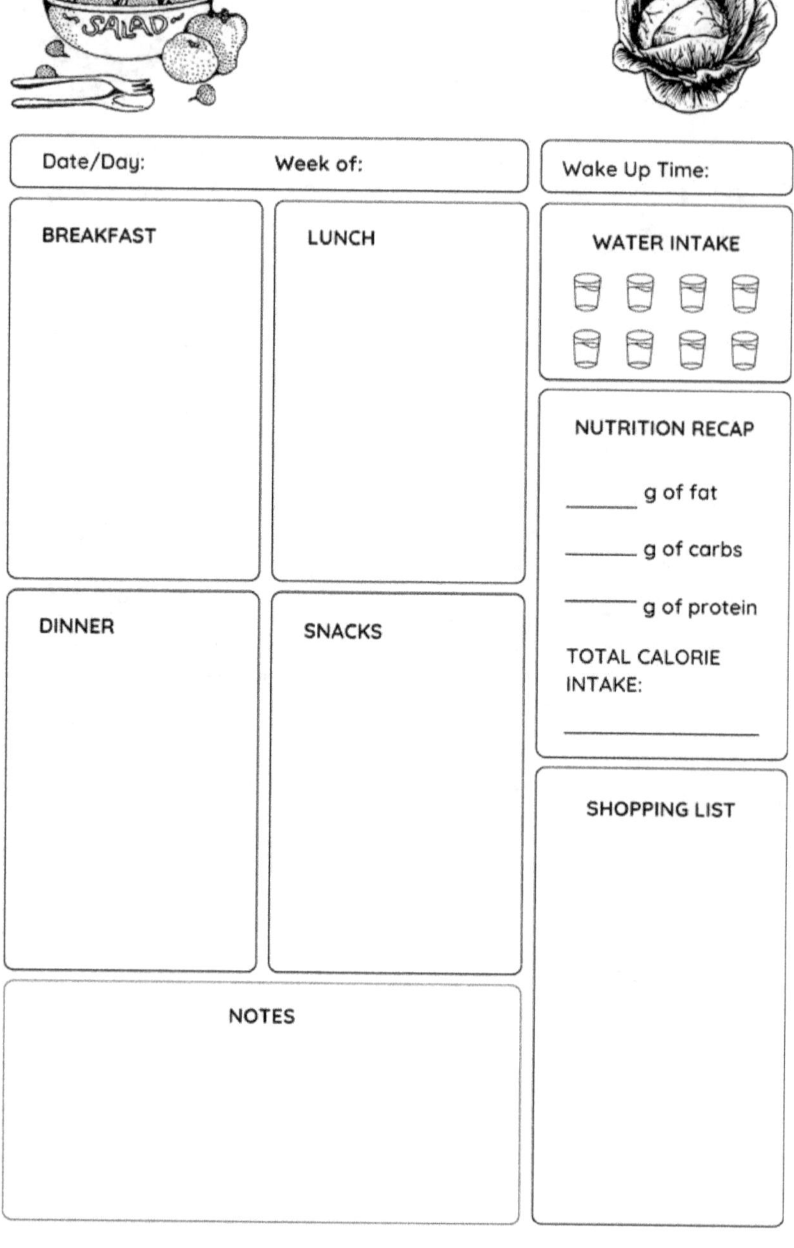

Date/Day:
Week of:
Wake Up Time:
BREAKFAST
LUNCH
WATER INTAKE
NUTRITION RECAP
_______ g of fat
_______ g of carbs
_______ g of protein
TOTAL CALORIE INTAKE:
DINNER
SNACKS
SHOPPING LIST
NOTES

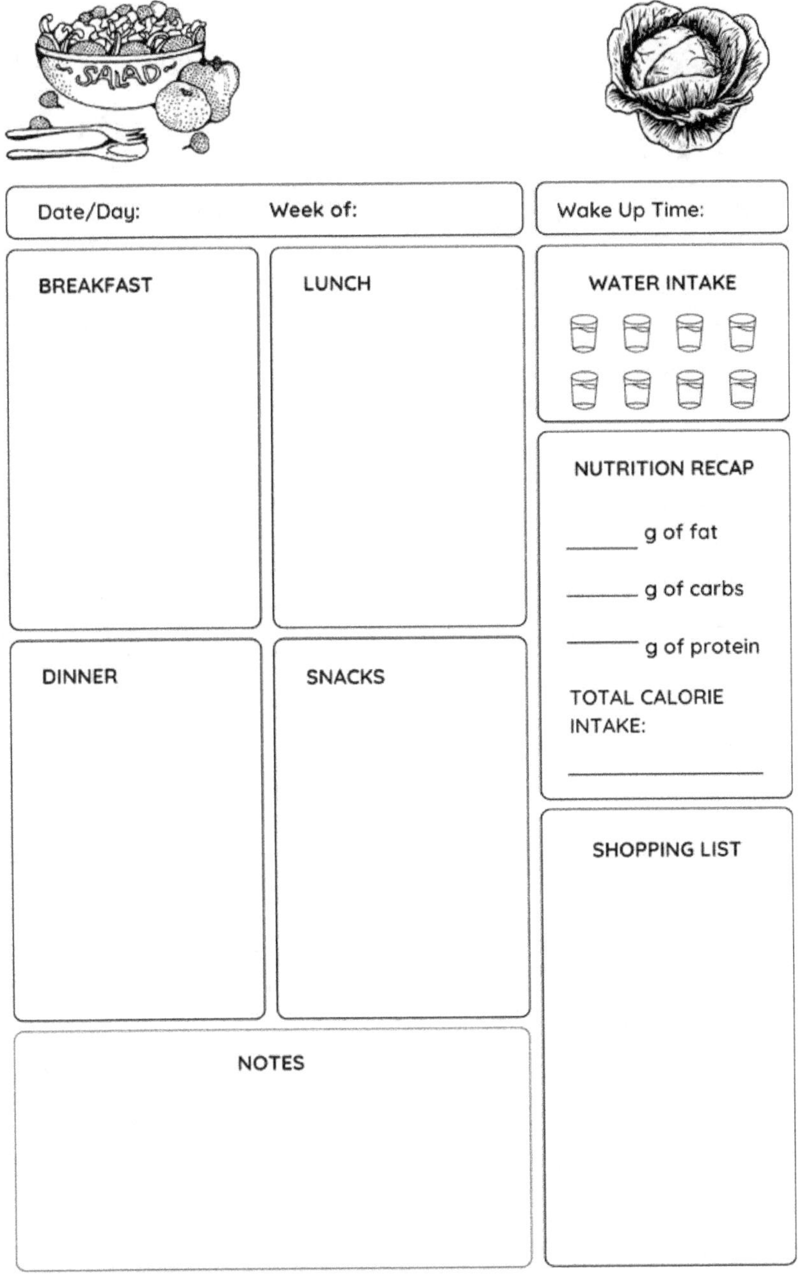

| Date/Day: | Week of: | Wake Up Time: |

BREAKFAST

LUNCH

WATER INTAKE

NUTRITION RECAP

_______ g of fat

_______ g of carbs

_______ g of protein

TOTAL CALORIE INTAKE:

DINNER

SNACKS

SHOPPING LIST

NOTES

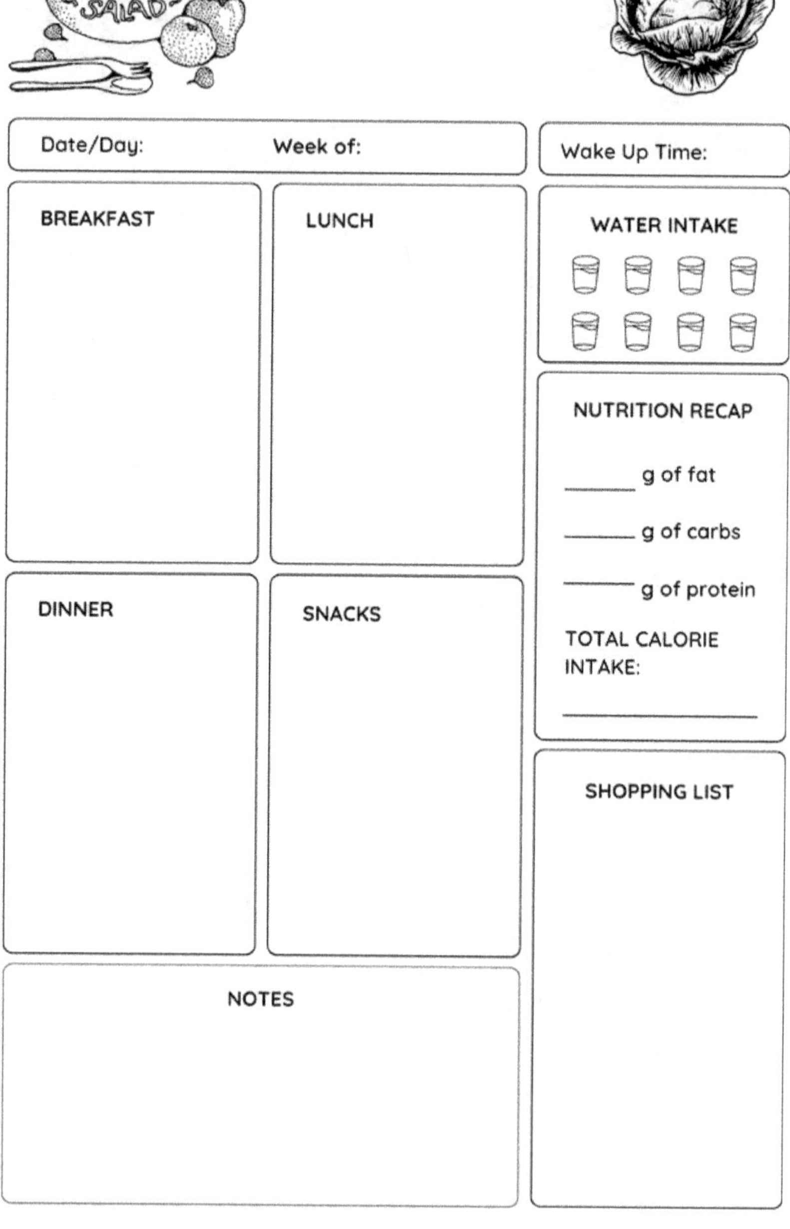

Date/Day:
Week of:
Wake Up Time:
BREAKFAST
LUNCH
WATER INTAKE
DINNER
SNACKS
NUTRITION RECAP
_______ g of fat
_______ g of carbs
_______ g of protein
TOTAL CALORIE INTAKE:
SHOPPING LIST
NOTES

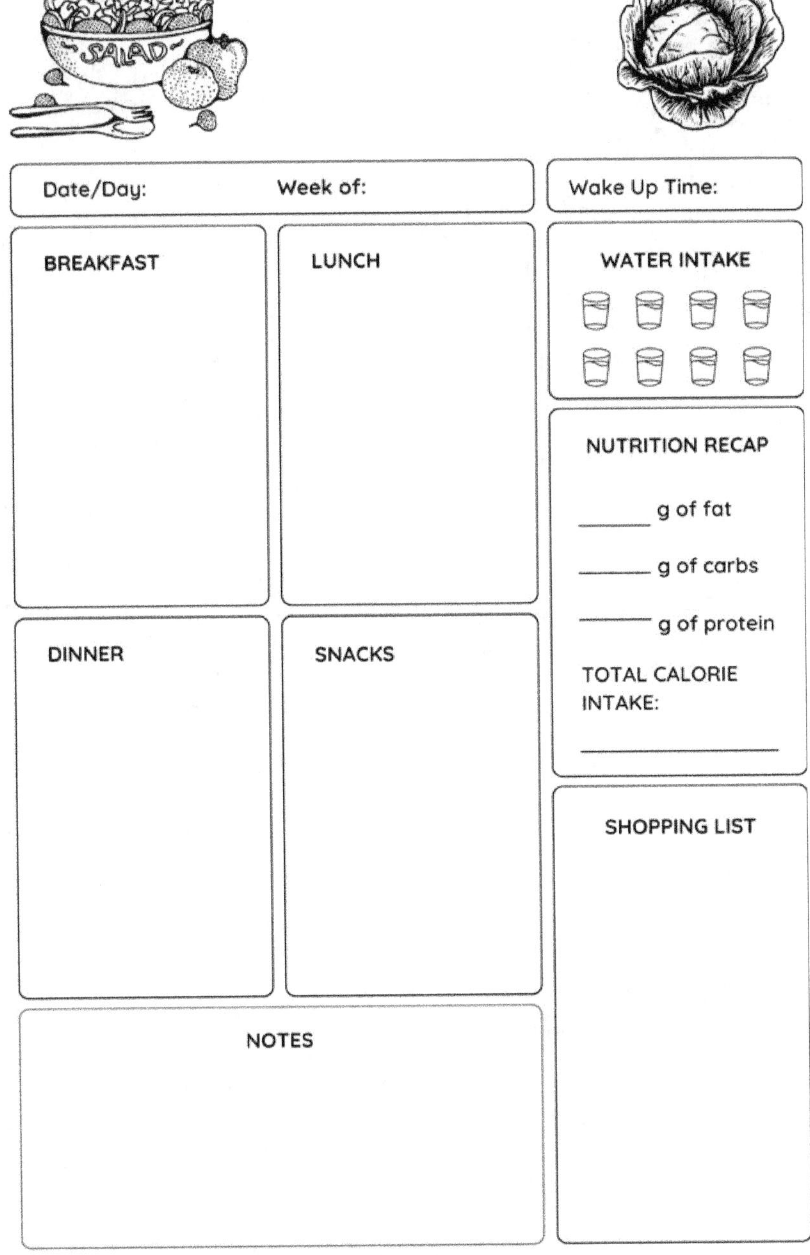

| Date/Day: | Week of: | Wake Up Time: |

BREAKFAST

LUNCH

WATER INTAKE

NUTRITION RECAP

_______ g of fat

_______ g of carbs

_______ g of protein

TOTAL CALORIE INTAKE:

DINNER

SNACKS

SHOPPING LIST

NOTES

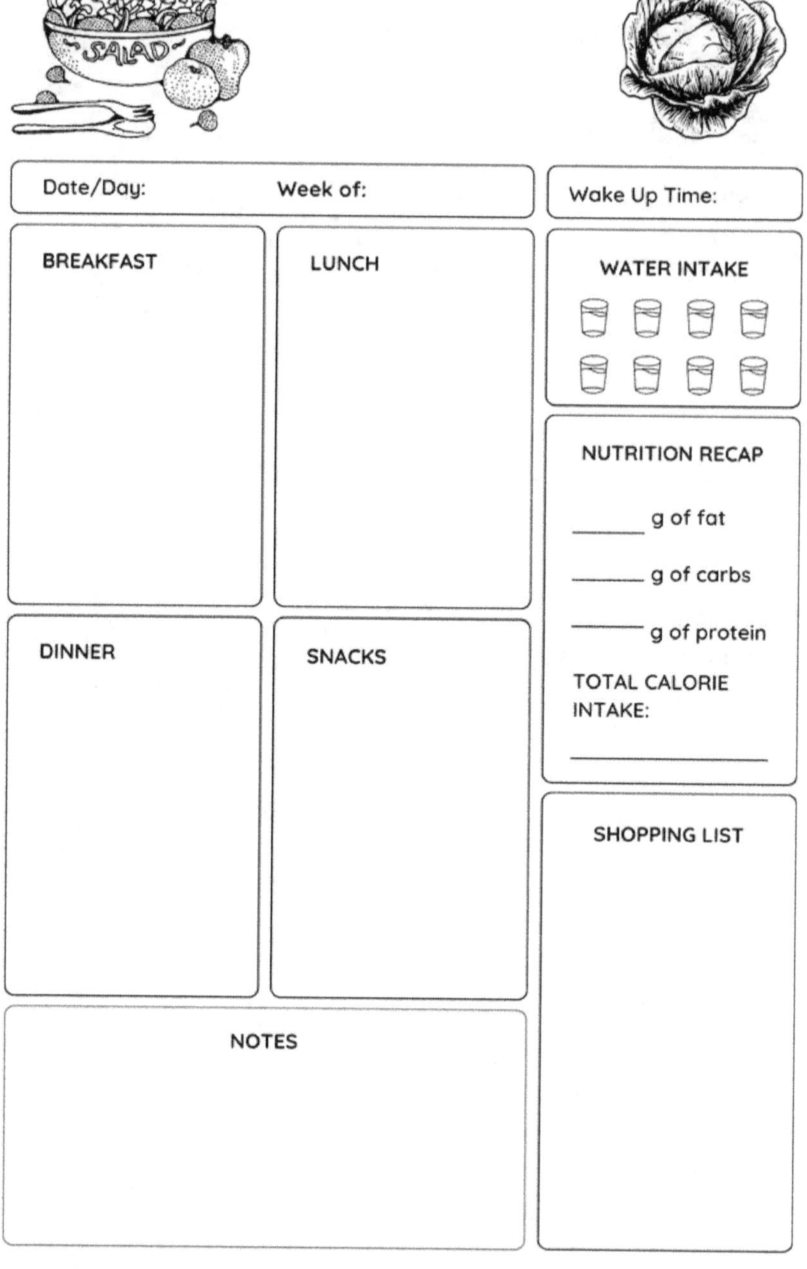

Date/Day:
Week of:
Wake Up Time:
BREAKFAST
LUNCH
WATER INTAKE
NUTRITION RECAP
_______ g of fat
_______ g of carbs
_______ g of protein
TOTAL CALORIE INTAKE:
DINNER
SNACKS
SHOPPING LIST
NOTES

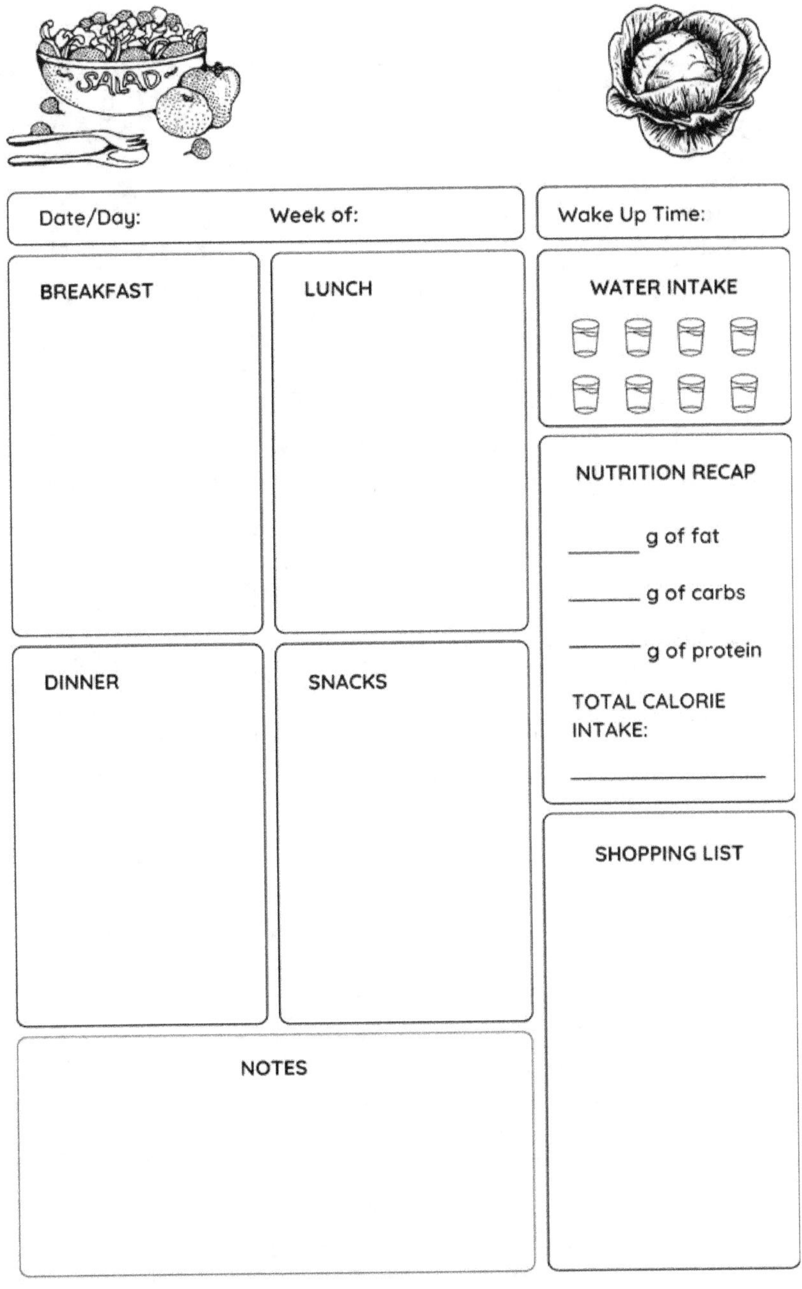

| Date/Day: | Week of: | Wake Up Time: |

BREAKFAST

LUNCH

WATER INTAKE

NUTRITION RECAP

_______ g of fat

_______ g of carbs

_______ g of protein

TOTAL CALORIE INTAKE:

____

DINNER

SNACKS

SHOPPING LIST

NOTES

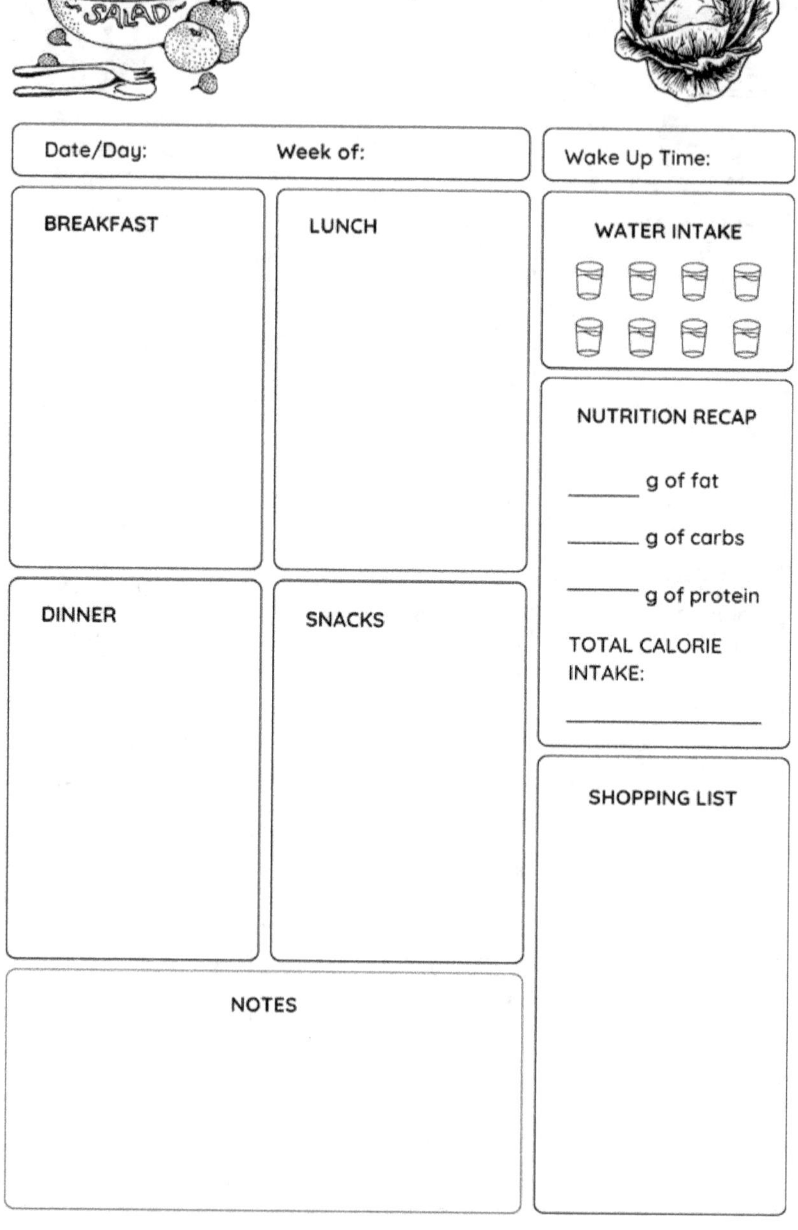

Date/Day:
Week of:
Wake Up Time:
BREAKFAST
LUNCH
WATER INTAKE
NUTRITION RECAP
_______ g of fat
_______ g of carbs
_______ g of protein
TOTAL CALORIE INTAKE:
DINNER
SNACKS
SHOPPING LIST
NOTES

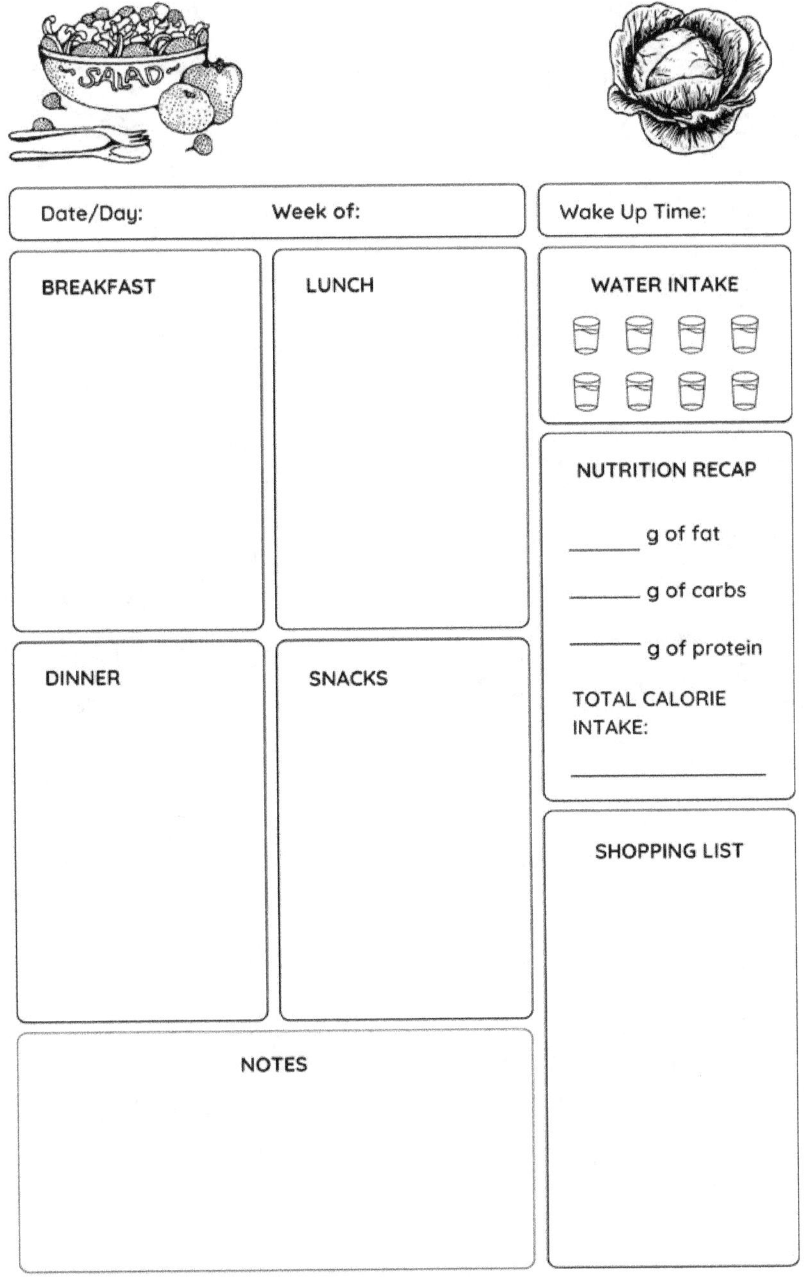

Date/Day: | Week of:

Wake Up Time:

BREAKFAST

LUNCH

WATER INTAKE

NUTRITION RECAP

_______ g of fat

_______ g of carbs

_______ g of protein

TOTAL CALORIE INTAKE:

DINNER

SNACKS

SHOPPING LIST

NOTES

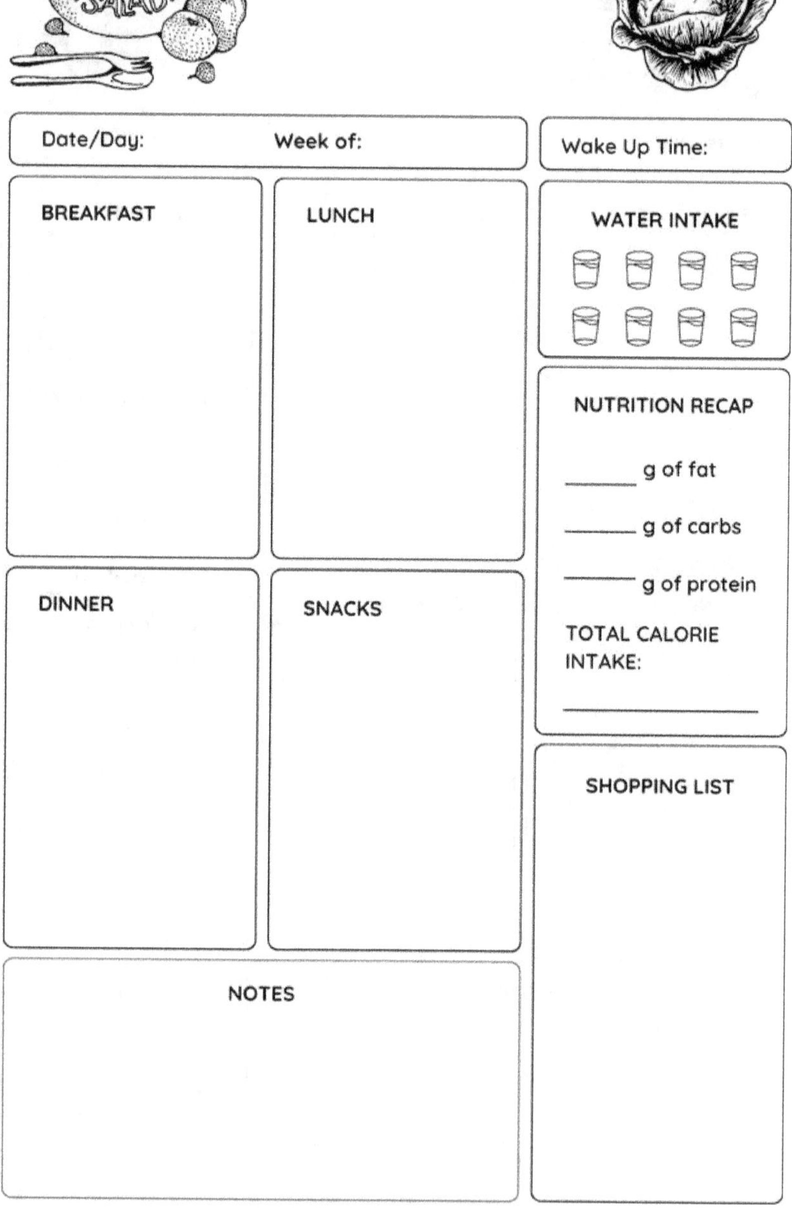

Date/Day:
Week of:
Wake Up Time:
BREAKFAST
LUNCH
WATER INTAKE
DINNER
SNACKS
NUTRITION RECAP
_______ g of fat
_______ g of carbs
_______ g of protein
TOTAL CALORIE INTAKE:
SHOPPING LIST
NOTES

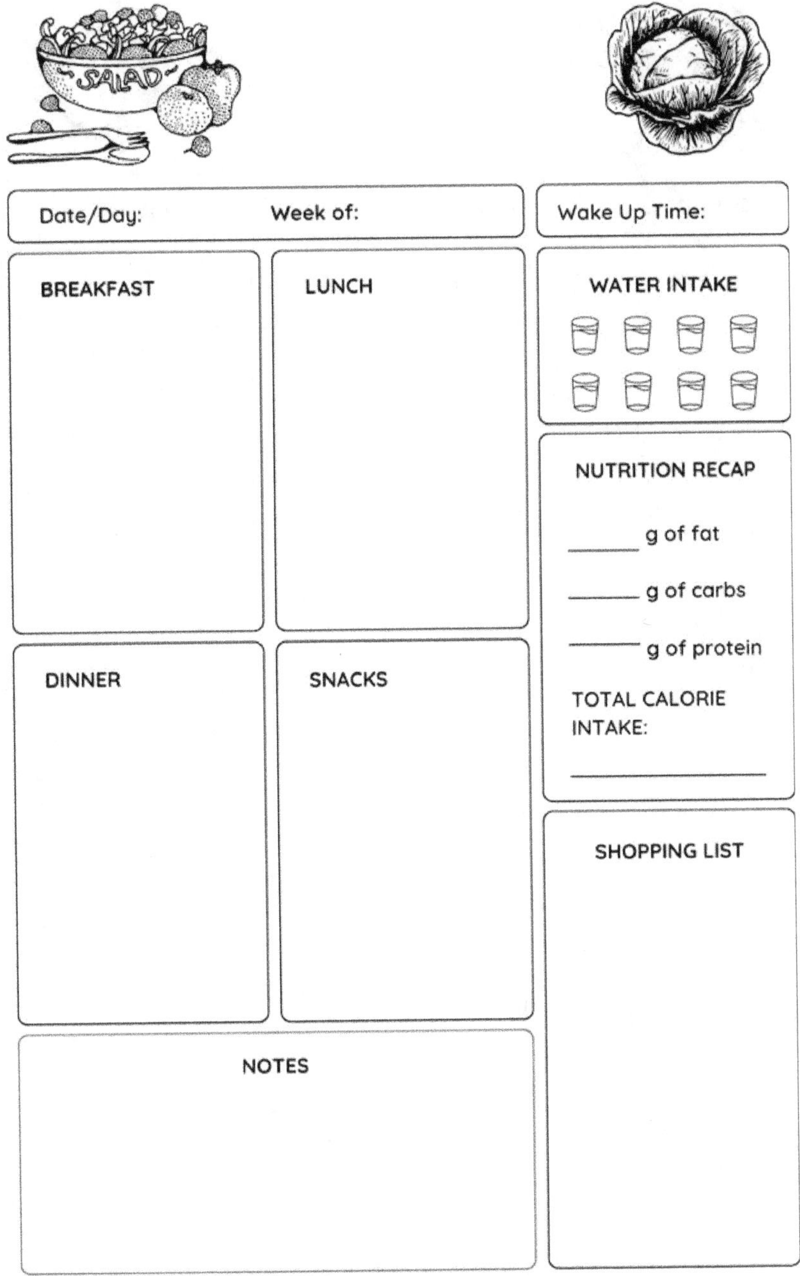

Date/Day: Week of:

Wake Up Time:

BREAKFAST

LUNCH

WATER INTAKE

NUTRITION RECAP

______ g of fat

______ g of carbs

______ g of protein

TOTAL CALORIE INTAKE:

DINNER

SNACKS

SHOPPING LIST

NOTES

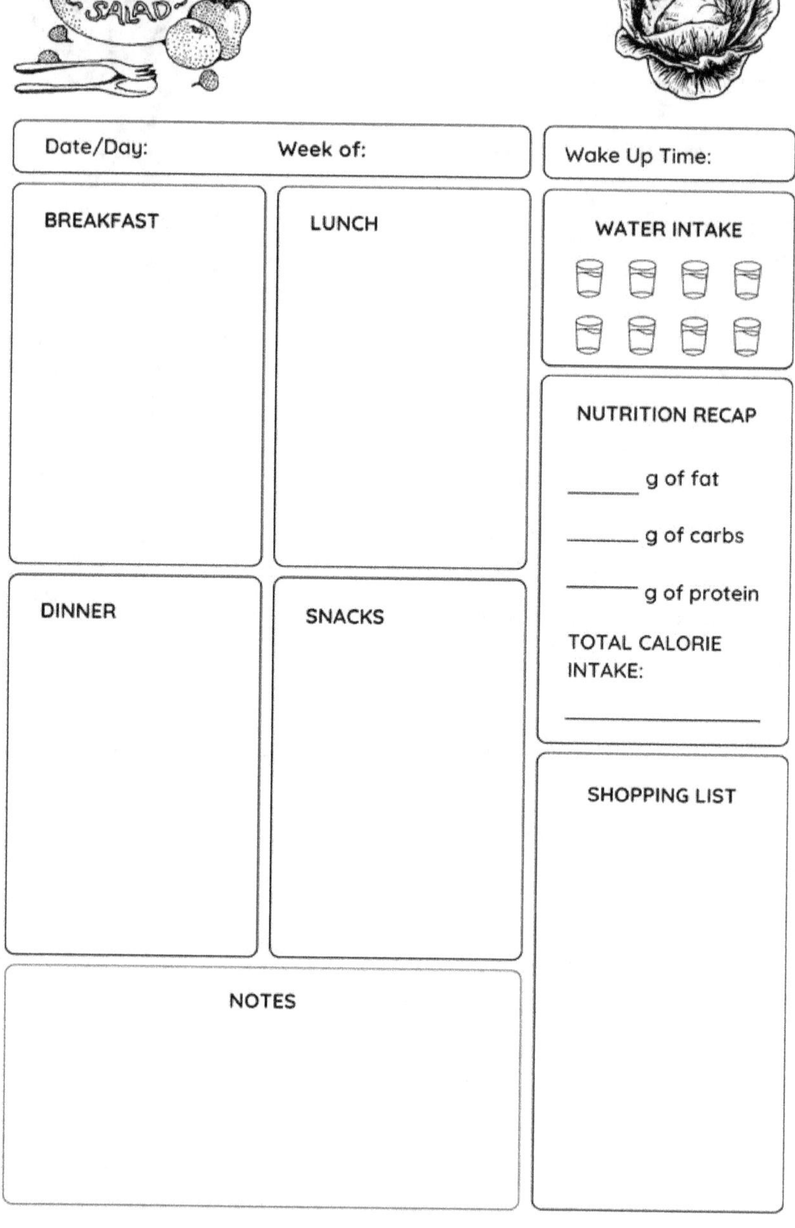

Date/Day:
Week of:
Wake Up Time:
BREAKFAST
LUNCH
WATER INTAKE
DINNER
SNACKS
NUTRITION RECAP
_______ g of fat
_______ g of carbs
_______ g of protein
TOTAL CALORIE INTAKE:
SHOPPING LIST
NOTES

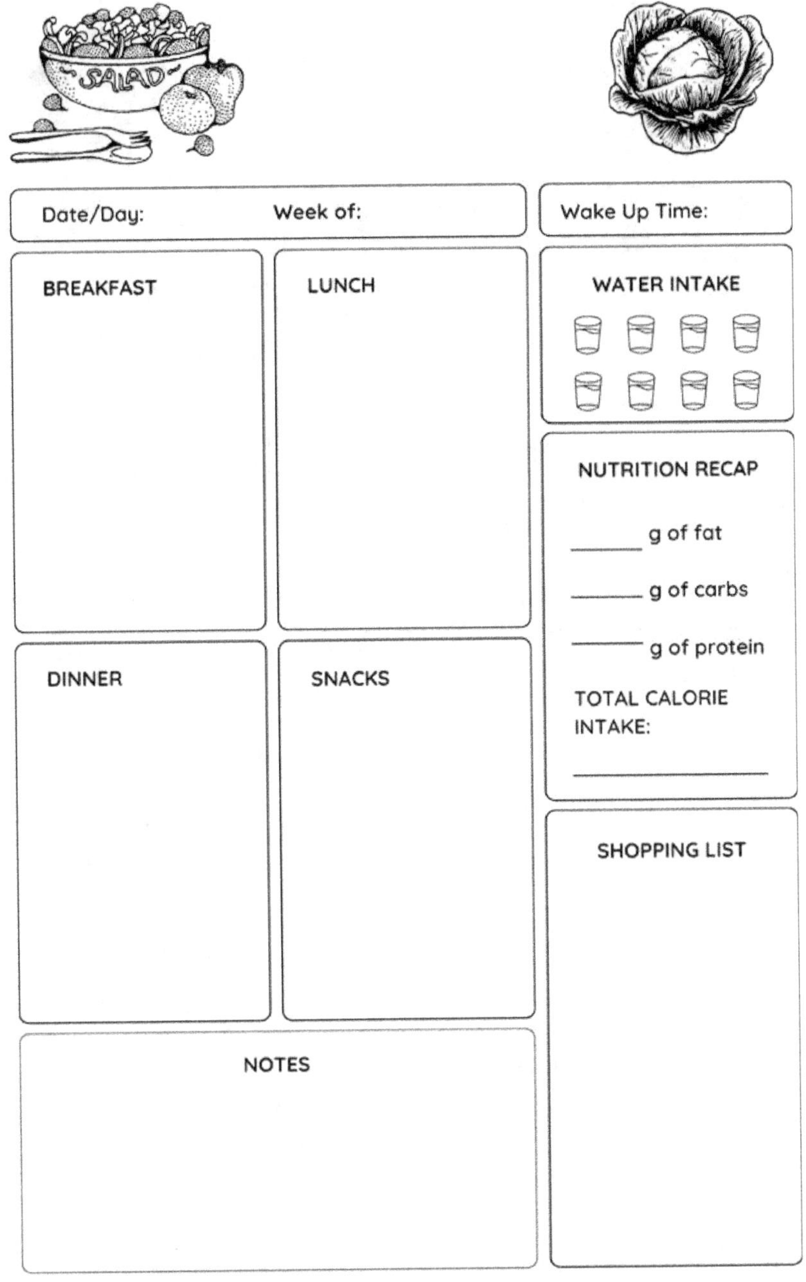

Date/Day: Week of: Wake Up Time:

BREAKFAST

LUNCH

WATER INTAKE

NUTRITION RECAP

_______ g of fat

_______ g of carbs

_______ g of protein

TOTAL CALORIE INTAKE:

____

DINNER

SNACKS

SHOPPING LIST

NOTES

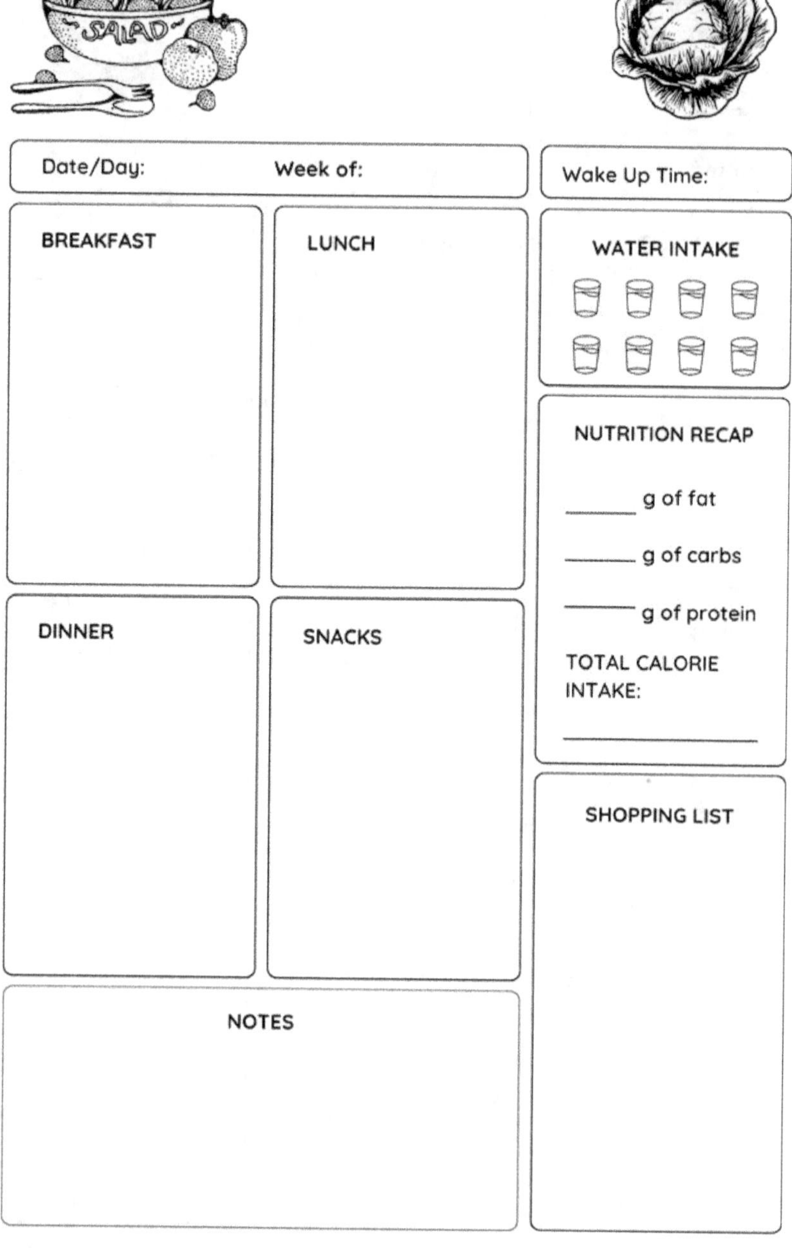
SALAD
Date/Day:
Week of:
Wake Up Time:
BREAKFAST
LUNCH
WATER INTAKE
NUTRITION RECAP
_______ g of fat
_______ g of carbs
_______ g of protein
TOTAL CALORIE INTAKE:
DINNER
SNACKS
SHOPPING LIST
NOTES

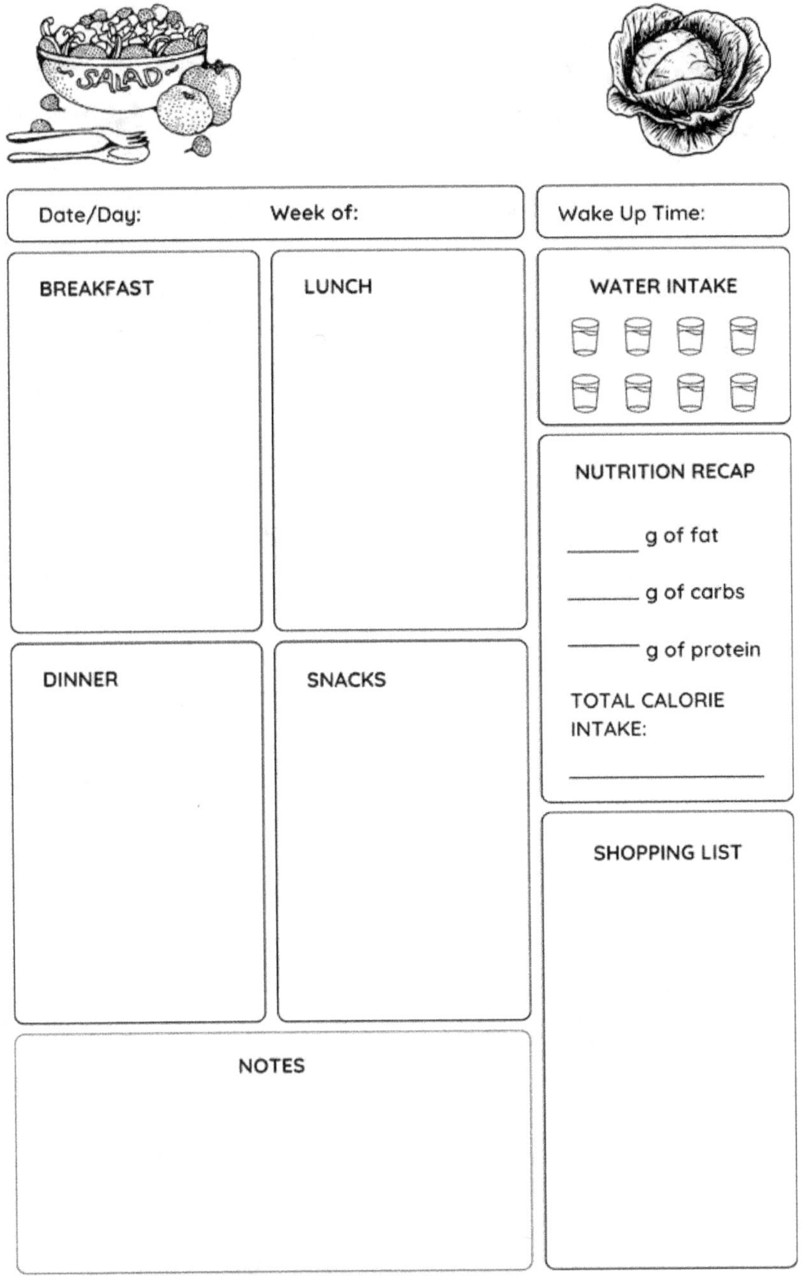

Date/Day: Week of:
Wake Up Time:
BREAKFAST
LUNCH
WATER INTAKE
NUTRITION RECAP
_______ g of fat
_______ g of carbs
_______ g of protein
TOTAL CALORIE INTAKE:
DINNER
SNACKS
SHOPPING LIST
NOTES

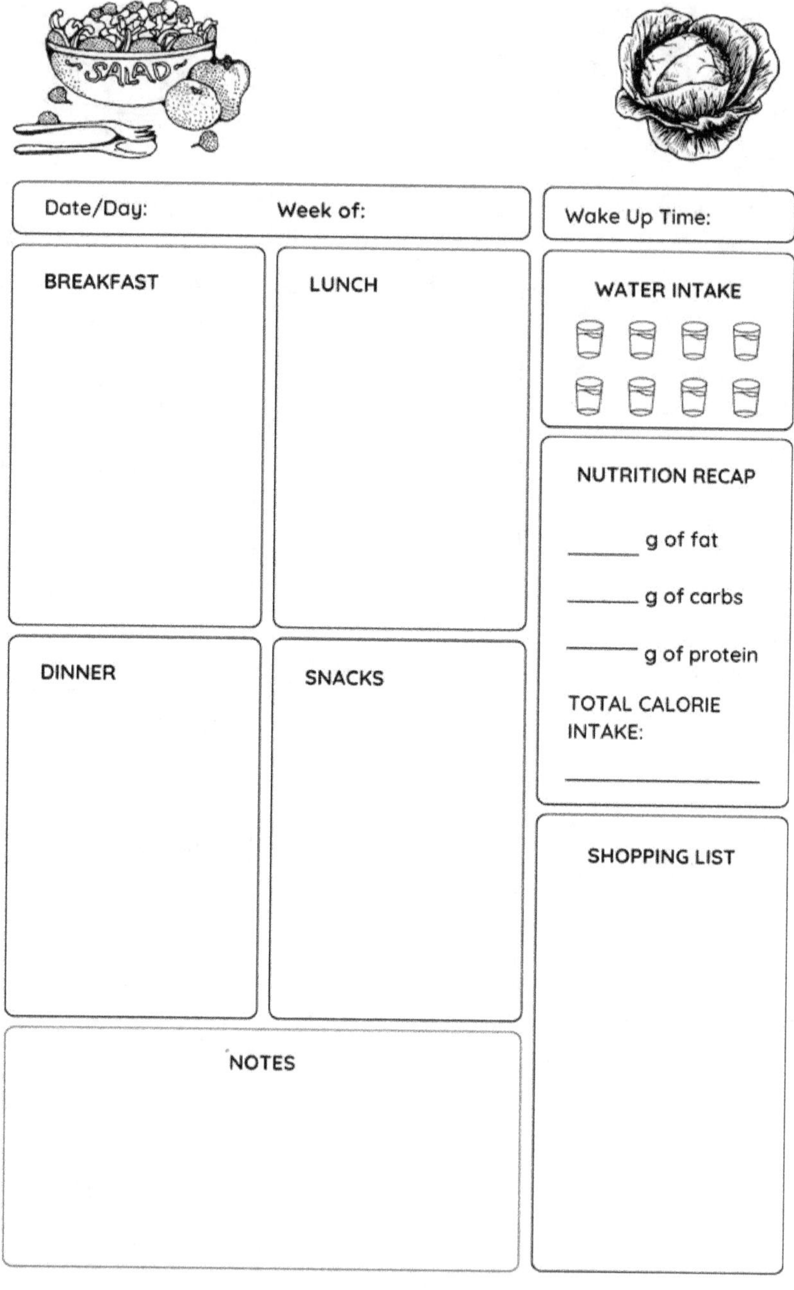

Date/Day: Week of:

Wake Up Time:

BREAKFAST

LUNCH

WATER INTAKE

NUTRITION RECAP

_______ g of fat

_______ g of carbs

_______ g of protein

TOTAL CALORIE INTAKE:

____

DINNER

SNACKS

SHOPPING LIST

NOTES

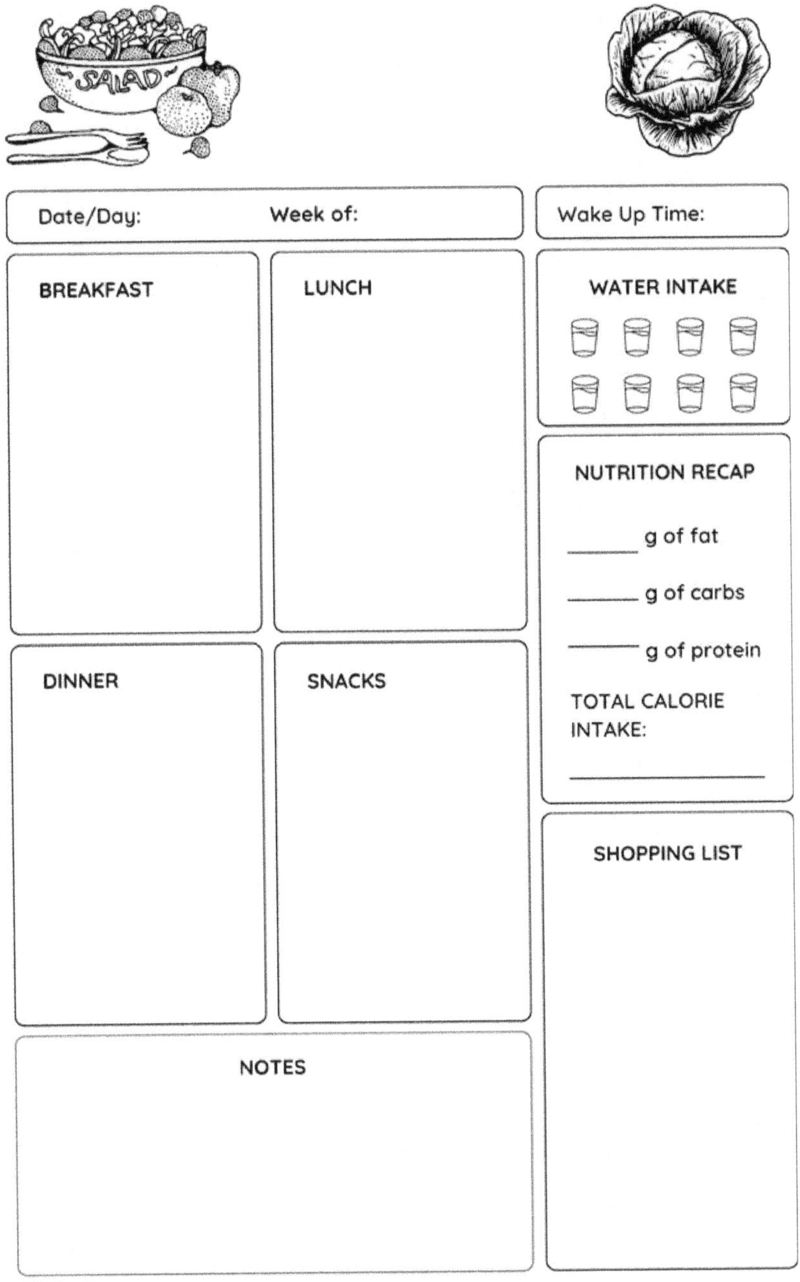

Date/Day:
Week of:
Wake Up Time:
BREAKFAST
LUNCH
WATER INTAKE
NUTRITION RECAP
_______ g of fat
_______ g of carbs
_______ g of protein
TOTAL CALORIE INTAKE:
____
DINNER
SNACKS
SHOPPING LIST
NOTES